The Consulting
Veterinary Nurse

The Consulting Veterinary Nurse

Nicola Ackerman
BSc(Hons) RVN CertSAN CertN ECC A1 V1 C-SQP

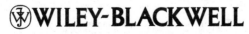
WILEY-BLACKWELL

A John Wiley & Sons, Ltd., Publication

This edition first published 2012 © 2012 by John Wiley & Sons, Ltd

Wiley-Blackwell is an imprint of John Wiley & Sons, Ltd, formed by the merger of Wiley's global Scientific, Technical and Medical business with Blackwell Publishing.

Registered office: John Wiley & Sons, Ltd, The Atrium, Southern Gate, Chichester, West Sussex, PO19 8SQ, UK

Editorial offices: 9600 Garsington Road, Oxford, OX4 2DQ, UK
The Atrium, Southern Gate, Chichester, West Sussex, PO19 8SQ, UK
2121 State Avenue, Ames, Iowa 50014-8300, USA

For details of our global editorial offices, for customer services and for information about how to apply for permission to reuse the copyright material in this book please see our website at www.wiley.com/wiley-blackwell.

Library of Congress Cataloging-in-Publication Data

Ackerman, Nicola.
    The consulting veterinary nurse / Nicola Ackerman.
        p. ; cm.
    Includes bibliographical references and index.
    ISBN 978-0-470-65514-6 (pbk. : alk. paper)   1. Veterinary nursing.
2. Pet medicine.   I. Title.
    [DNLM: 1. Animal Technicians–Great Britain.   2. Animal
Diseases–nursing–Great Britain.   3. Veterinary Medicine–Great Britain.
SF 774.5]
    SF774.5.A25 2012
    636.089–dc23
                                2012005127

A catalogue record for this book is available from the British Library.

Wiley also publishes its books in a variety of electronic formats. Some content that appears in print may not be available in electronic books.

Cover design by Meaden Creative.

Set in 10/12.5 pt Sabon by Toppan Best-set Premedia Limited

1   2012

Contents

Foreword

The Consulting Veterinary Nurse is a useful reference for all veterinary nurses who run clinics in their practice. The author, Nicola Ackerman, is an experienced Registered Veterinary Nurse and she has drawn on her knowledge to provide a comprehensive guide, which includes information on how to run efficient and effective well pet clinics and medical clinics.

The book contains a wealth of information on all aspects of running a clinic, including: how to provide clients and patients with an excellent level care; the answers to questions which clients frequently ask in a clinic; how to gather a patient's history; carrying out an examination and the necessary equipment for this – along with a list of common abbreviations. Nicola also discusses the role of the veterinary nurse and the consideration of nutritional and behavioral issues within the setting of a veterinary nurse-lead clinic.

This book will be a useful reference for both veterinary nurses who are experienced in running clinics and those who are just starting out.

Helen Farrant on behalf of the BVNA

Abbreviations

AAA	aromatic amino acids
ACE	angiotensin converting enzyme
ADH	antidiuretic hormone
ALA	alpha-linolenic acid
ALP	alkaline phosphatase
ALT	alanine aminotransferase
AMTRA	Animal Medicines Training Regulatory Authority
ARD	antibiotic-responsive diarrhoea
BCAA	branched-chain amino acids
BCS	body condition score
BER	basal energy requirement
BV	biological value
CHD	canine hip dysplasia
CHF	congestive heart failure
CRF	chronic renal failure
CS	chondroitin sulphate
DCM	dilated cardiomyopathy
DCP	dyschondroplasia
DER	daily energy requirement
DEXA	dual-energy radiographic absorptiometry
DHA	docosahexaenoic acid
DJD	degenerative joint disease
DM	dry matter
DMB	dry matter basis
DOD	developmental orthopaedic disorders
EAA	essential amino acids
ECG	electroencephalogram
EFA	essential fatty acids
EPA	eicosapentaenoic acid
EPI	Exocrine pancreatic insufficiency
FLUTD	feline lower urinary tract disease
FOS	fructo-oligosaccharides
GAG	glycoaminoglycan
GALT	gut-associated lymphoid tissue

GDV	gastric dilation–volvulus
GE	gross energy
GFR	glomerular filtration rate
GGT	gamma-glutamyl transpeptidase
HE	hepatic encephalopathy
IBD	inflammatory bowel disease
IBS	irritable bowel syndrome
IDDM	insulin-dependent diabetes mellitus
Ig	immunoglobulin
IRIS	International Renal Interest Society
MCS	muscle condition score
ME	metabolisable energy
MER	maintenance energy requirement
MTP	microsomal triglyceride transfer protein
NE	net energy
NFE	nitrogen-free extract
NIDDM	non-insulin-dependent diabetes mellitus
NRC	National Research Council
NSAID	non-steroidal anti-inflammatory drugs
NUVACS	National Unit for the Advancement of Veterinary Communication Skills
OA	osteoarthritis
OCD	osteochondrosis dissecans
PLE	protein-losing enteropathy
PSGAG	polysulphated glycoaminoglycan
PSS	portal systemic shunts
PUFA	polyunsaturated fatty acid
RAA	renin–angiotensin–aldosterone
RER	resting energy requirement
ROS	reactive oxygen species
RVN	registered veterinary nurse
SCFA	short-chain fatty acid
SG	specific gravity
SH	sodium hyaluronate
SIBO	small intestinal bacterial overgrowth
SQP	suitably qualified person
STT	Schirmer tear testing
TPN	total parenteral nutrition
VFA	volatile fatty acids
VLDL	very low-density lipoproteins
VSA	Veterinary Surgeons Act 1966

Introduction

The role of the veterinary nurse has evolved greatly, from being merely a kennel maid to a fee-earning regulated professional. Nurses have a vital role to play in the veterinary practice, in the offering of advice to clients, performing work in order for the veterinary surgeon to make a diagnosis, and in preventive healthcare.

For a nurse with a keen interest in consulting, this is an ideal opportunity to pursue the specialism that interests them while still being of use to the veterinary practice. Veterinary practices are businesses, and nurses that consult need to perform sufficient work in order to not only cover their costs and overheads, but also to make a profit. This is not necessarily through charging for nurse clinics, but through products sold, increasing footfall through the practice, helping with client loyalty and promoting compliance with veterinary advice.

Simplistically, nurse consultations create loyalty, are a better welfare choice and add to the commercial success of the business.

Veterinary nurses who fully utilise skills learnt during training are more likely to remain with the profession, and feel more valued members of the practice. Veterinary nurses are not 'mini-vets' and perform a completely different role to veterinary surgeons, though veterinary surgeons also undertake many roles that can be done by nurses, such as blood sampling and postoperative checks.

The purpose of this text is to act as a source of information for those veterinary nurses who undertake consultations, clinics and other initiatives such as puppy parties.

Acknowledgements

I would like to acknowledge all of the support from all of my family, friends and colleagues that has enabled me to complete this book. The role of the veterinary nurse has changed dramatically even within the time I have been practising, and I hope that this text will enable more nurses to become involved in consulting and expand their roles within veterinary practices.

I would therefore like to acknowledge all the veterinary nurses who have led the way in enabling veterinary nursing to become a recognised profession in its own right, both the RCVS VN Council and the BVNA.

Part I

The Role of the Nurse in the Veterinary Practice

1 Ethics

The role of the veterinary nurse has evolved into a regulated profession. A registered veterinary nurse (RVN) is regulated by the Royal College of Veterinary Surgeons under the Veterinary Surgeons Act 1966 (VSA). A solid understanding of this legislation is required in order to ensure that your actions are not only within the law but also in line with the professional code of conduct.

As a consulting nurse it is important to know your own limits, both to be within the law and not to exceed your own personal limitations. Under the VSA only veterinary surgeons are permitted to make a diagnosis. When examining an animal or answering an owner's questions, you must take care in the area of diagnosis. The veterinary nurse is permitted to inform the owner of the clinical symptoms that the animal is displaying, such as weight loss, increased thirst, tachypnoea, anaemia. You can discuss conditions that display these symptoms, and give guidance on what steps the owner needs to take next – for example, consultation with a veterinary surgeon. If it is likely that the animal will require further investigations, such as blood tests, the owner should be advised that this may occur in the veterinary consultation and the owner can prepare the animal if required; for example, they can pre-starve the patient rather than having to come back for an additional appointment.

Suitably qualified persons

It is useful for veterinary nurses to have the 'suitably qualified person' (SQP) qualification in order to prescribe and dispense appropriate medicines for animals. The SQP qualification is regulated by the Animal Medicines Training Regulatory Authority (AMTRA) and requires annual retention fees alongside continued professional development that has been approved by AMTRA. Many anthelmintics are prescription-only medicine (POM-VPS) or in the non-food animal (NFA-VPS) category, which means they can be prescribed by a veterinary nurse with the appropriate SQP qualification. It is necessary for a nurse who conducts clinics to

The Consulting Veterinary Nurse, First Edition. Nicola Ackerman.
© 2012 John Wiley & Sons, Ltd. Published 2012 by John Wiley & Sons, Ltd.

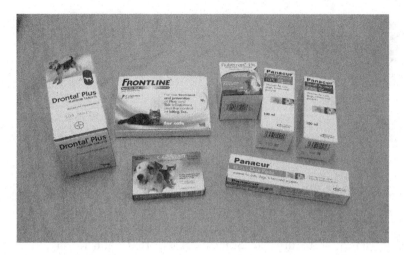

Figure 1.1 Example of anthelmintics that SQPs can prescribe.

hold this qualification, so that appropriate anthelmintics can be given without needing to consult the veterinary surgeon (Figure 1.1).

One of the roles of the veterinary nurse is to ensure compliance with recommendations given by the veterinary surgeon. Sometimes this can refer to medications, and you should confirm with the owner that they are able to administer the medications that have been prescribed. In some cases a different format of medication, such as liquid instead of tablets, can be helpful. These cases require not just an initialled change to the prescription, but a separate prescription that must be written by the veterinary surgeon.

When animals are presented to the veterinary nurse for a repeat of injectable medications a veterinary surgeon stills needs to be present in the building as you are administering the medication under veterinary direction. The veterinary surgeon should be in a position to intervene if required, even after they have prescribed the medication.

As an RVN is it vital to have personal indemnity insurance. RVNs are responsible for their own actions, and this includes any work undertaken within a consultation or clinic. Indemnity insurance for RVNs can be included under the veterinary practice's insurance policy for all staff, or as a personal policy for those who are self-employed. Self-employed locum nurses have to ensure that they are adequately insured.

During a consultation, the person conducting the consultation is responsible for the health and safety of all the people in the room; this includes the client. This means that if the client is hurt, even if by their own pet, the practice is responsible. Any injuries, such as bites or scratches, should be entered into the practice's Accident Book. It is therefore prudent to ask a colleague to restrain any animals that are not being adequately cooperative. If children are being unruly, you are within your rights to request the parent/guardian to ask their children to behave. If con-

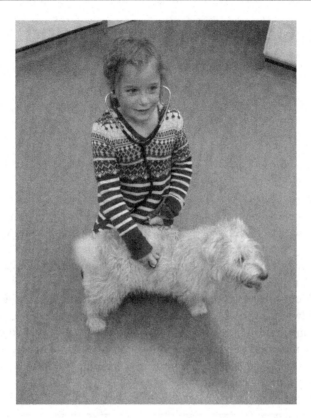

Figure 1.2 Entertainment for children can prove to be a useful distraction during lengthy consultations.

sultations are going to be lengthy, activities to keep children occupied can be a useful distraction. Pictures to colour in, or a pretend 'vet kit' with a stuffed toy, can be a great hit with younger children (Figure 1.2). The pictures that they draw or colour can be put up on the wall or notice board.

2 Consulting Room and Literature

When conducting their own nurse clinics or consultations, nurses need to portray themselves as professionals. This includes how and where the nursing consultations are held. Having to conduct a consultation in the waiting room or preparation room does not portray the person holding the consultation as professional. If you are conducting your own consultations then it is important to have a room dedicated for this purpose.

The nurses's consulting room, like a veterinary surgeon's consulting room, needs to be clean, tidy and fit for purpose. All of the equipment that you will require to conduct the consultation needs to be in working order and easily to hand (see Box 2.1). All other members of staff, especially receptionists, need to be made aware that during the specified block of time this consulting room is to be kept solely for the use of nurse consultants.

Box 2.1 Equipment required for the consulting room

- Microchip scanner and microchips
- Various types of nail clippers
- Bandaging materials
- Grooming combs and brushes
- Toothbrushes and paste
- Leaflets
- Pen, and paper to write on
- Slip lead
- Suture and staple removers
- Weighing scales
- Thermometer
- Vaseline
- Gloves
- Cotton wool
- Table cleaning disinfectants
- Hibiscrub
- Tape measure

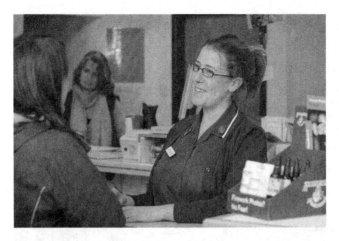

Figure 2.1   Always be happy to speak to clients in reception.

On many occasions clients turn up to the practice in person without an appointment, or telephone in wanting advice. You should always make an effort to speak to these clients; if it is not possible to speak to them immediately, you should offer to contact them later (Figure 2.1). Receptionists should take appropriate contact details and/or make an appointment for the client to bring their pet in to see you. The consulting veterinary nurse should appear as approachable as possible.

Environmental factors within the consulting room are also important. It is important for the room to have good ventilation and temperature control (Figure 2.2).

Some consultations may be lengthy – for example, an initial consultation for an obesity clinic. It is therefore important to have chairs in the consulting room, as some clients will prefer to sit down.

Literature

Most clients will find it difficult to remember everything that is said to them in the course of a consultation. It is helpful to give clients handouts on what you have been discussing, and in some cases to give specific written instructions. When clients walk out of the consultation room with information in hand, they have a perception that they have received better value for money than if they just walk out empty-handed. Clients who have received written instructions, either a handout or specific written instructions, are more likely to comply with the instructions given to them.

The literature that you decide to use in your consultations with clients needs to be of a high standard. There are two views of what types of literature should be used. One approach is to use only literature that is produced by the veterinary practice itself, with the practice's branding on it. In this case all the literature is in line with your practice policy, and you can be completely at ease with what is

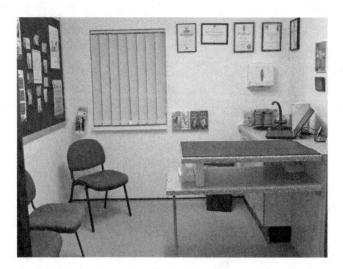

Figure 2.2   The consulting room needs to be clean and ventilated.

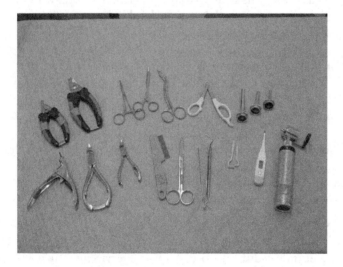

Figure 2.3   Examples of equipment required in a consulting room.

written there. The other approach is to use literature that is produced by manufacturing companies. This is generally well written and produced to a very high standard, but sometimes it is written around a specific product, rather than around a condition, which can be a disadvantage. Many pharmaceutical companies are now producing condition-specific literature, because of the restrictions on advertising of prescription-only veterinary medications (POM-V) directly to pet owners.

Any equipment you may need during the consultation needs to be present in the consulting room. All equipment needs to be clean and in working order. It can be useful to label equipment in order to designate it to each specific consulting room, in order to ensure that the required equipment is always to hand (Figure 2.3).

3 The Consultation

Several frameworks for consulting have been developed for medical education, but none has been developed specifically for veterinary use. There is considerable overlap between the two fields, so it was decided to adapt a widely used medical consultation model to the veterinary context, taking account of the likely differences between veterinary and medical consultations. The Cambridge-Calgary consulting model (Figure 3.1) has been adapted by the National Unit for the Advancement of Veterinary Communication Skills (NUVACS), and is therefore the most relevant to the veterinary profession.

Preparation

Before starting any consultation it is important to prepare adequately. Any equipment required for the consultation should be prepared (see Chapter 2) and the consulting room needs to be clean. You should read through the clinical history of the animal, as you need to be fully aware of any relevant previous history. Whether or not the consultation is about the previous clinical history of the animal, if you mention or ask how the animal has been since the incident, the client feels that you care about their pet. It is always worth checking vaccination status, last time of worming, and other parasite control. If any relevant comments have been noted in the clinical history, the client should be reminded about these. For example, if the veterinary surgeon has requested repeat blood sampling or a repeat clinical examination in a specified period of time, the client should be reminded about it. Make a note of the animal's name, sex and age, and use this information when talking to the client.

Your appearance is also a highly important factor in the client's perception of you. The nurse's uniform needs to be as clean as possible and hair should be kept tidy; long hair should be tied back. All staff members should wear name badges, which should be visible. Even though you tell the client your name at the time, many clients are stressed and do not remember many important facts, let alone the nurse's name. When writing down any future appointment times, write your

The Consulting Veterinary Nurse, First Edition. Nicola Ackerman.
© 2012 John Wiley & Sons, Ltd. Published 2012 by John Wiley & Sons, Ltd.

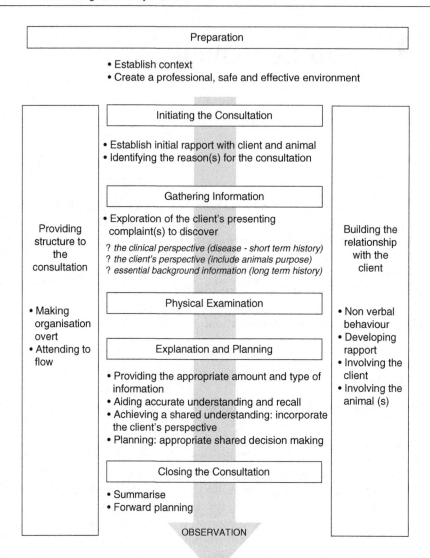

Figure 3.1   Adapted Cambridge-Calgary model of veterinary consultation skills.

name next to the time. Photographs of staff members can be useful for clients, and help to increase the recognition of the role of the veterinary nurse within the veterinary practice (Figure 3.2).

Initiating the consultation

The consultation should start with your confirming the name of the client when calling them through from the waiting area. Always introduce yourself, and

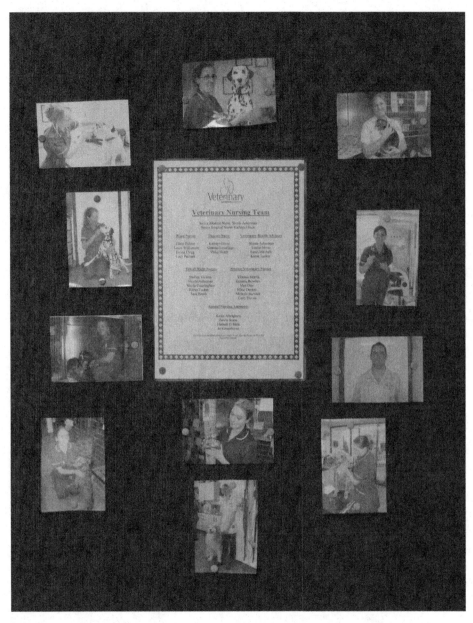

Figure 3.2 A display of the practice nurses and their roles can help to raise the recognition of the veterinary nurse.

confirm what the appointment is for. For example, 'Hello, my name is Nicola, I am your nurse for today. Have you brought Timmy for his blood test?' There are many occasions when the client will make an appointment for one cat, and then bring the other instead as the initial cat hasn't made it into the cat transport box. There are also occasions when the reason for the consultation can change, but this

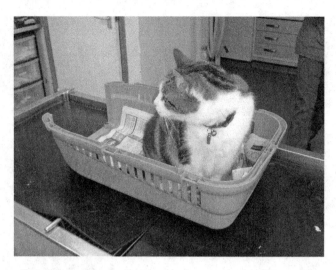

Figure 3.3   A cat less stressed in the bottom half of its transportation box.

only becomes apparent when the animal is presented. If there has been a delay in the starting time of the appointment, you should apologise for this. Clients (and pets) don't like to be kept waiting, and not acknowledging it can make the situation worse.

You should also acquaint themselves with the animal. Dogs should be patted and cats removed from transport baskets. Use of the pet's name is vital. If a cat is not willing to come out of its basket, removing the top half of the basket is helpful. The cat can then be examined in the bottom half of the basket, or lifted out on its blanket on to the consulting table (Figure 3.3). This is why cat owners are always recommended to purchase cat transport boxes that can be opened from the top.

This stage is very important for creating rapport with the client and their pet. Remember to use names, shake hands with the client, greet the pet and, most importantly, involve the pet. In order to create good rapport, veterinary nurses need to empathise with pet owners. Owners need to see, hear and feel these emotions from the practice as a whole, not just from the veterinary nurse that they see in the nurse consultations. In most cases they think of their pet as part of the family, and this special bond needs to be respected.

Information gathering

Background information can be gained from the clinical history, but in many cases additional information is required and is obtained through questioning. Many clients are more than happy to offer information, whether it is relevant or not, but sometimes you will need specific questioning in order to get the required information. Both open and closed questioning should be used when conducting a con-

---

Box 3.1   Open and closed questioning

Open questioning

An open question can be defined as one that is likely to receive a long answer (not just yes or no).

Although any question can receive a long answer, open questions deliberately seek longer answers, and are the opposite of closed questions.

Open questions have the following characteristics:

- They ask the respondent to think and reflect.
- They give you *opinions* and *feelings*.
- They hand control of the conversation to the respondent.

Closed questioning

A common definition is that a closed question can be answered with either a single word or a short phrase. Thus 'How old are you?' and 'Where do you live?' are closed questions. A more limiting definition is that a closed question can be answered with either yes or no.

Closed questions have the following characteristics:

- They give you *facts*.
- They are easy to answer.
- They are quick to answer.
- They keep control of the conversation with the questioner.

Box 3.2   Effective listening

Good listening skills are an essential part of communication and have many functions:

- Seek clarification
- Take notes
- Avoid distractions
- Use pauses and silences
- Restate and summarise

---

sultation, as they will provide different types of answers (see Box 3.1). Questioning also helps provide information on the client's expectations, concerns, wants and needs. It allows you to demonstrate your professionalism and knowledge, while helping to build rapport and show empathy. Questions also help to give you time to think and time to focus. Ensure that you show genuine interest in what the client is saying; listen to what the client is saying and if necessary repeat what they are saying back to them in order to confirm details (Box 3.2).

This is a very important stage of the consultation, and one that is often overlooked or not fully completed. Sometimes when the consultation has finished the client often asks, '. . . and another thing'. This is an indication that questioning was not sufficiently thorough in the early stage of the consultation.

In some cases the client will ask for multiple procedures to be completed, or will have a very long list of questions. Your job is to find out what all of the client's concerns are and then prioritise which are the most important, to you as a veterinary professional and to the client. What you feel is the most important factor and what the client feels is the most important may be two different things. For example, the client may feel that having the pet's nails clipped is what they have presented their pet for, and this is the most important thing to be done in the consultation. You, however, may feel that the animals's dramatic weight loss and polydipsia are the most important factors to be considered. In this situation you need to ensure the client understands why you feel that these factors need to be prioritised over the nail clipping.

If the client has a long list of non-emergency questions or procedures, the consulting nurse and the client need to agree on which things are to be completed first. A subsequent appointment can be made on another day in order to complete the rest. This must be done in agreement with the client, and they must understand why some things are being deferred to another day, for the following reasons:

- Insufficient time to correctly cover all the items that the client wishes
- Too much information for the client to retain in one appointment
- The pet becoming stressed (e.g. at having all the mats combed out of its hair in one session)
- To aid in compliance.

For example, if you want to demonstrate to a client how to brush a dog's teeth, in the first consultation you can introduce the concept of the toothpaste or gel; the second consultation is to ensure that the client is managing stage 1 and is ready to move on to stage 2.

Physical examination

When initiating the physical examination it is important to be aware of the clinical history. If the animal is known to have a tender abdomen, or arthritic joints, it is important not to exacerbate any discomfort. With larger dogs, or those that do not like being on the consulting table, the physical examination can be conducted on the floor.

While carrying out the clinical examination it is important to talk through with the client what you are doing and looking for. Many clients comment that the veterinary surgeon only gave their pet a quick check over, or didn't actually examine it. In fact the pet was probably given a full clinical examination, but the owner was not aware of what the veterinary surgeon was doing. What the owner perceived as the veterinary surgeon fussing the dog, was actually them checking for lumps and bumps. When checking for lumps and bumps, check whether the client is aware of any; some lumps are small and may not be noticeable to you. Talk your way through the examination, starting from the top and systematically working backwards. Having a set routine for the clinical examination will help to ensure that things are not missed out.

Start by looking at the symmetry of the head and jaw. This is important when animals are presented with dental disease, as lumps or bumps on the jawbone can be an indicator of tooth root problems. Any nasal discharge should be noted, along with colour and whether a lateral or bilateral discharge is present. When examining the eyes, the size of the pupils and symmetry between the two eyes should be examined (Table 3.1). The conjunctiva surrounding the eye should be examined in order to check for infection, and any discharge from the eye should be noted. Tear overflow, and the staining of the fur that will be seen when checking puppies (Figure 3.4), should be discussed with the client. Ears should be checked, looking for discharge, general wax and dirt. Examination of the mouth will really depend on the animal's cooperation of the. If the animal is known to be difficult to handle,

Table 3.1 Possible underlying cause of anisocoria (unequal size of the pupils)

Nervous system causes	Ocular causes
Head trauma	Anterior uveitis (inflammation of a portion of the eye)
Disorders of the optic nerve, the primary nerve to the eye	Glaucoma (increased pressure in the eye)
Disorders of the oculomotor nerve, a cranial nerve that provides muscle sense and movement of the eye	Iris muscle abnormalities
Diseases of the cerebellum, an area of the brain	Eye cancer
Disorders of the optic tract, a bundle of nerve fibres associated with the eye	Medications that change the function of the pupil
	Spastic pupil syndrome

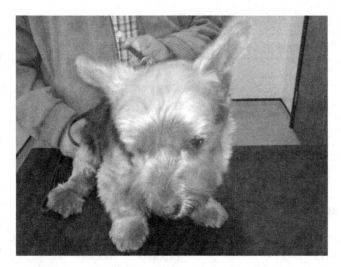

Figure 3.4 Tear overflow in a dog.

in some circumstances asking the owner to lift the animal's lip up so that you can look at the teeth can be appropriate. If any disease is present then it should be noted and graded. The level of gingivitis, plaque and calculus should be noted.

When feeling down the animal's neck and shoulders, the lymph nodes should be checked. If they are palpable this needs to be noted and referred to the veterinary surgeon. The condition of the coat and skin need to be assessed, and checked for parasites. Nail length should be noted.

Part of the examination should also include the heart rate, respiratory rate and temperature. The overall condition of the animal should be noted, e.g. body condition score (BCS), muscle condition score (MCS), weight, hydration status (see Box 3.3 and Table 3.2).

Explanation and planning

Once all the information has been gathered and the animal examined, you need to explain your findings to the owner and a mutually agreed plan needs to be made. When explaining and planning the next steps it is important to convey the

---

Box 3.3   Signs that can be used to assess hydration levels

- Tenting of skin
- Sunken eyes
- Haemoconcentration of blood constituents
- Ability or inability to sweat
- Quantity of urine produced
- Blood pressure
- Capillary refill time (CRT)
- Dryness of mucous membranes

Table 3.2   Assessing levels of dehydration in an animal

Percentage of dehydration	Clinical signs
<5%	No obvious outward signs Concentrated urine
5–8%	Slightly prolonged CRT Slight tenting of the skin Mucous membranes feel tacky Third eyelid visible
8–10%	Sunken eyes Prolonged CRT Obvious tenting of the skin
10–12%	Oliguria Tented skin remains in place Clinical shock can be experienced
>12%	Progressive shock Coma and death

CRT, capillary refill time.

information in a form that the client understands. This can be oral or written, and in some cases educational DVDs can be provided. Some points will need to be reiterated, and some relayed in a different form that will enable the owner to fully understand the information that is being conveyed. When planning the next step the owner must be in agreement with the decisions that are being made and must be able to comply with the instructions given. There are three parties involved in making any plans: the veterinary profession, the client and the pet. All parties need to be in agreement in order to make a plan work. The owner may agree to daily tableting, but the pet may not be in complete agreement with this plan and therefore complications can occur.

Breaking down information into 'digestible' chunks can be helpful for the owner. In lengthy consultations it can be useful to ask the owner if they want to take notes – have a pen and paper ready in order to allow them to do so. It is important to ask the client if they can foresee any challenges of implementing this plan at home, as they might completely agree with what should be done, but may not be able to actually do it.

Closing the consultation

When closing the consultation the aim is to summarise the decisions that have been agreed on, and to arrange future appointments. It can also be useful to confirm that the owner is happy with any instructions for any medications that have been dispensed or diets recommended. Make sure the client has details of how to contact you by phone or e-mail, and also write your name down again. Many people will still forget what you initially told them, as they are understandably worried about their pet.

In all consultations, remember:

- Show courtesy and respect both to the client and to their pet.
- Provide solutions: even if this means having to refer the problem on to someone else, it is part of the pathway to providing a solution. Don't say 'I don't know' in relation to a specific problem, but turn the statement around to 'Let me find out for you', or 'Let's see what we can do'.
- Keep your word: if you say you will contact the owner in a couple of days, ensure that you do.
- Ask if there is anything else that you can do for the client. If the information-gathering stage of the consultation has been completed correctly then the client will usually say no. This gives them the feeling that all of their original expectations for the consultation have been met.

Compliance

Compliance is achieved when the owner fully understands what is required, and is able to undertake these requirements. Compliance has three beneficiaries:

- The pet (its health and welfare is increased)
- The owner (being able to have a happier, healthier pet)
- The practice (increasing client service, profits and increases in staff motivation).

Compliance can break down, and this can lead to less healthy pets, and fewer bonded clients. This can occur for a number of different reasons, mainly due to lack of understanding. Many clients do not understand the nature of their pet's disease or the requirement for continued long-term treatment, or may misunderstand what the veterinary professional has told them. In some cases the owner can be too embarrassed to ask the veterinary surgeon for further clarification. These cases tend to present as the owner stating that they felt that the pet seemed better, unsure of what the term 'chronic' meant, and that they felt or understood that just one course of the treatment was required. Few clients actually state cost as a factor in the breakdown of compliance. Apathy can be a major cause of compliance breakdown, but good support and client education on the importance of why medications should be given, or weight loss occur, can help to reduce apathy in pet owners.

Ensuring that all pets newly diagnosed with a disease have a follow-on appointment with a veterinary nurse a few days later is a really good protocol to instigate. The follow-up can be either in person or on the telephone if the owner is unable to attend. During these few days the client will have thought of a few questions, many of which they may feel are too trivial to ask the veterinary surgeon. Ultimately, this system will dramatically aid in increasing compliance (see Box 3.4).

Box 3.4   Measures commonly used to aid in increasing compliance

- Client education (client meetings, websites)
- Printed or written instructions (leaflets, handouts, written notes or emails)
- Follow-up calls, re-examination appointments, nurse clinics
- Identifying if the client would like additional clarification.

4 Diagnostic Clinics

Part of the veterinary nurse's role is to aid the veterinary surgeon in gathering data by collecting samples for diagnostic procedures. The nurse can carry out procedures such as blood sampling, blood pressure monitoring, Schirmer tear testing, skin sampling and urinalysis. Nurses are not permitted to make a diagnosis themselves, but are adequately trained in the preparation of the animal and the collection of samples so that the veterinary surgeon can make a diagnosis.

Blood sampling

Routine sampling for many conditions can be done by the veterinary nurse within the nursing consultation. Examples include repeat sampling for fructosamine levels in diabetic patients, haematology for chemotherapy patients and biochemistry parameters for renal patients. When taking samples it is important to agree whether or not to have the owner present during the procedure. Many owners will expect to remain while you take the sample; some will not want to be present, but they need to be aware of the option. You should also inform the owner that it is essential to clip any hair away from the sampling site in order to prevent infection; aseptic preparation of the site is required. If the animal requires more than one site to be clipped it is important to inform the owner of the reasons for this. Communication is exceptionally important in all nursing clinics and consultations, and owners like to be aware at all times of things that affect their pet.

Before taking the sample it is important to confirm that the owner understands why it is being taken. If it is a repeat procedure the owner may already be fully aware, but if the veterinary surgeon has requested sampling to be done in a subsequent nurse consultation, the owner may require clarification. Information about when the animal received medication, or if and when it was fed, need to be obtained. This consultation is also a good opportunity to weigh and condition score (BCS) the animal. In some cases this appointment may be the owner's only point of contact with a veterinary professional for the few months in between prescription or other veterinary checks. If the animal is suffering from a particular

The Consulting Veterinary Nurse, First Edition. Nicola Ackerman.
© 2012 John Wiley & Sons, Ltd. Published 2012 by John Wiley & Sons, Ltd.

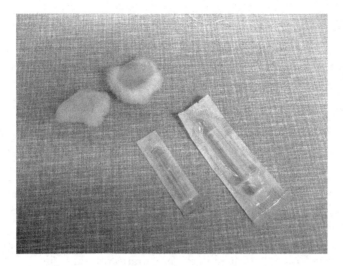

Figure 4.1 Equipment required for blood sampling.

condition, it is also a good opportunity to question the owner on the animal's overall condition, water intake, urine output, food intake, exercise tolerance and general demeanour.

Ensure that all materials required for blood sampling are prepared before bringing the client into the consulting room (Figure 4.1). All blood tubes should be labelled, and slides for haematology identified. When taking bloods for any haematological analysis, blood films should always be produced. If you are doing the sampling in the consulting room with the client present you will need a competent assistant in order to restrain the animal; always remember to introduce your colleague to the client.

It is important to note on the animal's clinical history where you took the sample from, and whether or not it was a stressed sampling. Blood samples taken from stressed cats will have an increased neutrophil count and stress hyperglycaemia. If the veterinary surgeon is not present when the sample is taken they will not be aware that the animal was stressed, and this can alter their interpretation of the results. Always ensure that the correct blood sampling tubes have been used for the types of tests that are to be performed, and for the laboratory that the samples are to be sent to.

Blood pressure monitoring

Routine blood pressure monitoring should be done in all patients suffering from renal disease, cardiac disease and diabetes, as well as all patients in the senior (mature) age category. It should ideally be done in the presence of the owner, as animals, especially cats, tend to be calmer when their owner is present. Cat owners should be encouraged to bring a blanket that the cat normally sits on at home, as

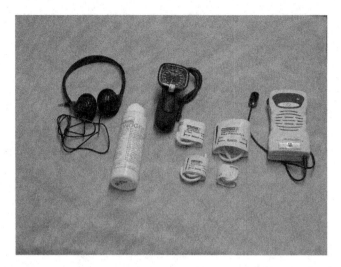

Figure 4.2 Equipment required for blood pressure measurement.

this will help the cat to relax more. Most cat owners tend to put these in the cat's travelling basket anyway. It is important to allow the cat to come out of the basket without dragging it out (alternatively, remove the top of its travel box), and for dogs to roam freely around the consulting room before monitoring the blood pressure.

All required equipment should be prepared beforehand (Figure 4.2). The cuff you will need to use should be pre-measured just before use, and the size used recorded on the clinical history. If different cuff sizes are used then different readings will be obtained. The secret here is to use the same cuff and site if you wish to monitor a patient long term. The cuff size is determined by the circumference of the limb on which it will be placed. For cats and dogs, the ratio of cuff width to limb circumference should be about 40%. If in between cuff sizes, round up. After placement, the cuff should not be so loose that it can be rotated over the site or so tight as to obstruct venous return. If it does not stay connected when inflated, select the next larger size cuff. A perfect fit will be with the self-attached loops just over the felt but not beyond.

The use of clippers to remove hair from distal to the carpal stopper pad should be avoided as this can inadvertently increase the blood pressure as a stress response in cats. Instead, wiping the area with surgical spirit and then rubbing ultrasound gel well into the hair works just as effectively. In order to remove any stress response to the noise created by the Doppler probe, headphones can be used. If these are not available, the noise should be turned off, the probe positioned, and then the volume slowly increased until the pulse is audible. (Figure 4.3).

All animals will react to the increasing pressure exerted by the cuff, and therefore the first reading should always be discarded, as it will be artificially elevated. Different sources will state different methods of finding a final measurement. Some recommend taking five readings and taking an average of the five, some suggest taking the third reading; personally, I repeat the process until three readings that

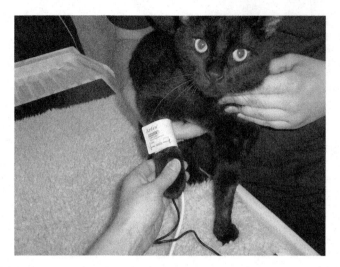

Figure 4.3   Cats should be minimally restrained for blood pressure monitoring.

are similar (within 5 mmHg) are recorded. Excess gel should be wiped from the animal, and the owner should be advised that it is not harmful if the animal licks any of it. The result, the cuff sized used and the location where the cuff was placed should all be recorded on the pet's clinical records.

Blood pressure monitoring is a useful diagnostic tool that should be used in many areas in veterinary practice. It is a good prognostic indicator for animals in a critical condition. The Doppler probes are also very useful for monitoring heart rate in small patients, such as rabbits, hamsters or birds, during general anaesthesia.

Urinalysis

The analysis of urine is a simple everyday task that can provide an excellent insight into the health of the patient. Specific gravity (SG) should be determined on every sample with use of a refractometer. When carrying out microscopy it is important not just to note whether there were crystals present but also the evidence of casts, cells and microorganisms.

Sample collection

The easiest and most commonly used method of collecting a sample is a free flow or voided sample. Collecting a midstream overnight sample is the best for routine urinalysis, as it gives the best indication of the true composition of urine.

The nature of the specific condition being investigated for will dictate what part of the sample is required. When collecting a sample for urethral plugs, uroliths

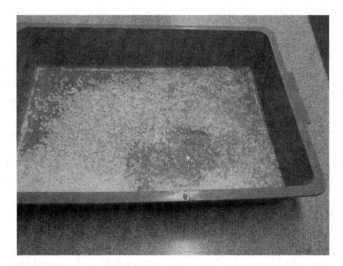

Figure 4.4   Non-absorbent cat litter.

and bacteria, the first part of the stream is the best. The end of the stream is the most appropriate to collect for examination for prostatic disease, haemorrhage or sediment analysis, because the sediment or haemorrhage collects on the floor of the bladder. Nearly all voided samples in cats are collected in a litter tray with non-absorbent litter, and these can prove to be invaluable in the treatment of urinary system problems (Figure 4.4).

Manual expression is an excellent method of sample collection, although it is dependent on the bladder being full. Excessive force on the bladder can cause haematuria, and potentially a ruptured bladder. Sterile samples for bacterial cultures can be obtained directly from the bladder by cystocentesis or via a urinary catheter. These two methods of collection are preferred; immediate analysis of the sample can often be performed in house.

Catheterisation of the bladder needs to be done aseptically in order to prevent introduction of bacteria into the bladder. Extreme care must be taken when placing the urinary catheter, otherwise traumatic damage to the lining of the urethra can occur, which will increase the number of erythrocytes and epithelial cells in the collected sample. Cystocentesis must also be performed aseptically and avoids the secretions and debris of the lower urinary tract. Iatrogenic haemorrhage can occur and should be considered when examining the sediment on microscopy. If ultrasonography is to be done as part of the diagnostic work-up, it should be performed before cystocentesis, as sampling can cause artefacts on the bladder wall that can be identified on the ultrasound scan.

Sample preservation

Many urine samples are refrigerated prior to analysis, as this process can slow down the degeneration of cells in the sample, the dissolution of casts (especially

Table 4.1 Examples of chemical preservatives for urinalysis

Chemical preservative	Analysis type	Comments
Boric acid	Bacteriology	Normally provided in commercial sample bottles
Formalin	Sediment. Kills bacteria and will alter protein results	1–2 mL formalin to 15 mL urine
Thymol	Biochemistry (except glucose) and sediment. Kills bacteria	Preserves urine for 24 hours
Toluene or hydrochloric acid	Biochemistry	Use a very thin layer over the surface of the sample

important in alkaline urine), and the bacterial conversion of urea to ammonia that will in turn cause a pH increase. It is this conversion and thus pH elevation that causes phosphates to precipitate out into the sample as triple phosphate (struvite) crystals. Refrigeration of the sample will also cause a change in the SG of the sample, and can interfere with some of the chemical reactions on the reagent strip. All refrigerated samples should therefore be brought up to room temperature before chemical analysis.

Chemical preservation of urine should be used if refrigeration is not possible (see Table 4.1).

Examination of urine

Gross examination

Visual inspection

Visual analysis of urine is the basic form of examination that should be performed first. The colour of the sample should be assessed, along with the turbidity (cloudiness). The transparency of the urine can be described as clear, cloudy or flocculent.

- Normal cat and dog urine should be **clear**, i.e. transparent.
- Equine and rabbit urine is **cloudy**, due to calcium carbonate crystals. Cloudy samples are those described as those containing large particles that usually yield large amounts of sediment when centrifuged.
- **Flocculent** samples contain suspended particles sufficiently large to be seen with the naked eye.

Samples that produce a small amount of white foam when shaken can contain large amounts of protein; the foam will remain longer than normal. Yellow-greenish foam indicates the presence of bile pigments in the sample (Figure 4.5).

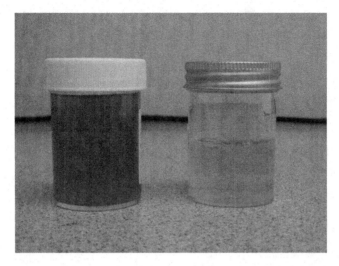

Figure 4.5 Macroscopic examination of urine should be performed and results noted.

Odour

The odour of a urine sample is not a diagnostic method, but sometimes be helpful. A sweet, fruity smell can indicate ketones, significant in diabetes mellitus.

Specific gravity

The SG is a measurement of the concentration of the urine. It is vital that this measurement is always taken when performing urinalysis using a refractometer. The concentration of the urine can also be a reflection of the renal function of the animal. A wide range of urine SG can be encountered in healthy animals – from 1.001 to over 1.075 for dogs and 1.001 to over 1.085 for cats. Values typically encountered for normally hydrated individuals are likely to be in the range 1.015–1.045 for dogs and 1.035–1.060 for cats. Failure to produce more concentrated urine in the presence of dehydration can indicate renal insufficiency (kidney disease).

Dipstick analysis

The sample should always be inverted before dipstick analysis, and it should be at room temperature. Dipstick analysis usually gives a qualitative guide to the levels of glucose, protein, blood, haemoglobin, ketones and bilirubin, although different sticks contain different analysis pads. Dipsticks designed for the human market may also measure SG, but this measurement is not accurate, and a refractometer should therefore be used (Figure 4.6)

The pH of the urine cannot be accurately measured with a dipstick. Results measured visually are not quantitative, and are open to interpretation by the

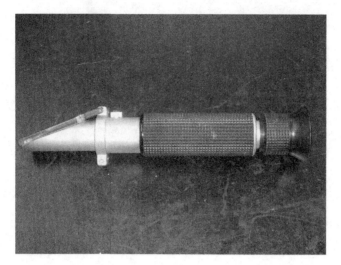

Figure 4.6 Use of refractometer for measurement of urine specific gravity.

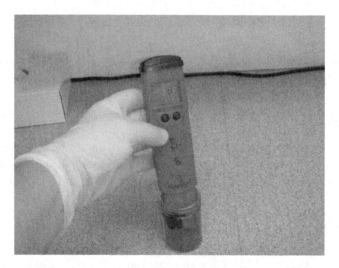

Figure 4.7 pH electrode used for urinalysis.

person performing the test. A pH meter should be used in order to obtain an accurate measurement of the urine pH. These meters are inexpensive and easy to use (Figure 4.7). If urine is being monitored for pH changes it is particularly important to use a pH meter, especially if you are checking pH to see if dose rates of acidifiers or alkalinisers should be altered.

Urine pH will alter throughout the day, especially urine formed after eating, which will be more alkaline. Dogs that have no access to food overnight will have more acidic urine in the morning. In order to reduce anomalies in urine pH, serial measurements can be taken throughout the day, in a similar format to blood glucose curves.

Schirmer tear testing

Schirmer tear testing (STT) should be a used as both a diagnostic tool and in screening programmes (see Box 4.1). Veterinary nurses are in an ideal position to aid in the instigation of screening programmes. Predisposed breeds that can be targeted for screening include cocker spaniels, bulldogs, West Highland white terriers, lhaso apsos, shih tzus, pugs and pekingese.

Box 4.1   Indications for the use of STT as a diagnostic tool

- Assessment of normal tear production
- Chronic mucoid epiphora
- Chronic pigmentary keratitis
- Epiphora

The prepackaged sterile strips are removed from the packaging and the notched end is placed in the lower conjunctival fornix. The strip should be in direct contact with the cornea. It is important not to touch the notched end, as lipids from your skin can affect the movement of the dye (Figure 4.8). The eye is held closed and the strip allowed to remain in place for exactly 1 minute. If convenient, both eyes may be tested at the same time. The strip is then removed and the tear production is measured and recorded using the standard measurement on the package. Normal dogs should secrete 15 mm or more in one minute. Topical anaesthetic is not used for this test as it is designed to measure the response of the eye to an irritant.

There are three layers to the tear film, and the STT only measures the aqueous middle layer; deficiency of the inner mucin layer or the outer lipid layer may also cause corneal irritation and opacity.

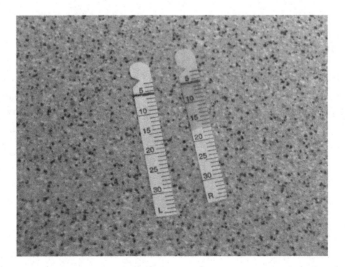

Figure 4.8   Schirmer tear testing strips.

Faecal analysis

A faecal examination involves the microscopic evaluation of faeces (see Box 4.2). This test is indicated for pets with diarrhoea, straining, inability to maintain an ideal body condition score (BCS), lack of appetite or vomiting. In many cases samples are sent to external laboratories for analysis, but microscopic examination can be done within the veterinary practice.

Faecal smears can be easily taken and examined microscopically. Their purpose is to provide a quick and simple but relatively insensitive method for demonstrating helminth infection and identifying the eggs and larvae present. This technique is non-quantitative (i.e. it does not provide a specific number of eggs or larvae) and it is a very insensitive method unless there is a very high helminth burden. Interpretations should be made carefully, as debris can overlie eggs or larvae.

Box 4.2   Materials required for microscopy of faecal smears

- Microscope slides
- Coverslips
- Saline solution (0.85%) or water
- Microscope
- Spatula to spread out the faecal matter

Worm egg counts using the modified McMaster egg count technique are commonly performed. Other methods of confirming parasite presence can be achieved by flotation methods, larval culture, Baermann techniques or faecal sedimentation techniques.

A full faecal analysis will identify whether there are any undigested materials such as fats and proteins in the faeces; this can show whether there is a possible maldigestion or absorption disorder.

Pooled samples

In many cases shedding of eggs and larvae can be intermittent and therefore pooled samples are required in order to make a positive identification of a causal agent. Normally faecal samples are collected over a 3 day period and all samples are sent to the laboratory for analysis.

5 Marketing

Marketing is an important element in the success of all ventures in veterinary practice. Marketing is about building relationships and the development of your practice brand – your name, your staff, your premises and your practice values for quality, courtesy, care, honesty, reliability, availability and value for money. It also includes the knowledge and professionalism of the staff.

Having a marketing plan for the year ahead can help to concentrate efforts on each specific event at the appropriate time. Annual events such as National Rabbit Week, Arthritis Month, Pet Smile Month, etc., can be included in the yearly plan. Events that are open to the public help to raise the practice profile, as well as educating people about how to care for animals (Figure 5.1). Seasonal trends such as the increased risk of chocolate poisonings at Christmas and Easter, and seasonal newsletters (e.g. to advise tortoise owners about hibernation, sent out during late summer or early autumn) can also be added to the calendar (Table 5.1).

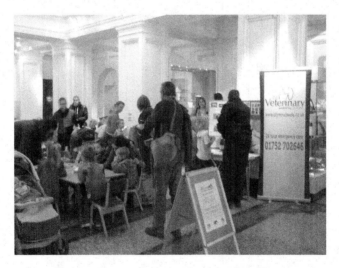

Figure 5.1 Public events not only help to educate the public but also raise the practice profile.

The Consulting Veterinary Nurse, First Edition. Nicola Ackerman.
© 2012 John Wiley & Sons, Ltd. Published 2012 by John Wiley & Sons, Ltd.

Table 5.1 Calendar of events. Light grey blocks represent planning and implementing stages, dark blocks represent the doing stages

	Jan	Feb	March	Apr	May	June	July	Aug	Sept	Oct	Nov	Dec
Seasonal events			Chocolate poisoning display in reception	National Rabbit Week (NB date changes from year to year)				Tortoise hibernation letter				Chocolate poisoning display in reception
Puppy clinics												
Obesity clinics												
Dental clinics												

All events and/or clinics need to be carefully planned and researched, with all required resources gathered before implementing. At least 2 months lead-in is required for most events. The first month is for planning what you want to do. If the plan is to launch a specific clinic, you need to decide on the protocol for what is going to be included in the clinic, which animals are to be included (a specific age group, for instance) and what literature is going to be used all. The second month is for instructing the other members of staff about what is planned and to ensure that all necessary training is completed before the desired start date.

6 Named Nurse and Protocol Writing

Named nurse

It can be difficult for clients to contact the right person in a veterinary practice when they need to. Having a specific point of contact really helps to put the owner's mind at ease and saves them a lot of worry. A named nurse who is knowledgeable about the case details and knows the client is an ideal point of contact.

Many questions that clients have can be answered by a veterinary nurse. For those that can't be, the nurse can find out by asking the veterinary surgeon, and relaying the answers back to the owner. Of course, there may come a point where the client needs to be referred directly to the veterinary surgeon.

A nurse who has a specific interest in certain medical problems, or owns a pet that has undergone similar surgery to the client's, may be just as knowledgeable as the veterinary surgeon. This nurse does not necessarily need to be the clinic nurse, but it does help, as these nurses are the ones who have the most contact with the owner. Little things such as what litter to use in the tray postoperatively, or describing over the phone how to administer medications, make a lot of difference to owners. These are the things that veterinary nurses are most adept at doing. They are also the things that help to increase owner compliance.

Statistics tells us that if you are told a lot of information at once you will only truly remember three or four details. So if you are discharging a medical case back to the client they will remember that their cat is OK, what you did to it, what is wrong with it and what medication it is on. If you give them a lot more information – it has to be on a specific diet, when their next appointment is, any clinical signs that they need to look out for, that the cat needs to lose weight, etc. – you can imagine that remembering your name is probably one of the last things that they will think of. But they will probably phone you to ask whether their pet needs to start the tablets tonight or tomorrow, even though you told them twice. Always write your name down for clients, with a contact phone number. If possible, have business cards with your name and contact details, and write everything down on a discharge sheet. Always ask owners if they have any questions, and tell them that you don't mind if they phone you later about something they thought of on the way home, or about any problems they encounter.

The Consulting Veterinary Nurse, First Edition. Nicola Ackerman.
© 2012 John Wiley & Sons, Ltd. Published 2012 by John Wiley & Sons, Ltd.

If you only work part time, tell the clients this. They don't expect you to be there 24/7, they just need to know when they can contact you without having to chase you.

Having a named nurse is now a must for all chronic cases. Owner compliance is important from an animal welfare point of view, but also from a business point of view. Just sending an animal home with a pot of tablets, and telling the owner to bring it back when the pot is empty, is a poor standard of practice. If the owner is only able to administer one tablet in a week, instead of two a day, they will not come back for months. If you notice that a certain client hasn't been in for their medication in a while, why not contact them and check that everything is OK? Clients like to see that you and the practice are taking an interest in their animal.

Veterinary nursing is a service-related industry, involved in the care of animals. Providing a service that can help increase the well-being and welfare of animals in our care is a must.

Protocols

There will be times when the named nurse or clinic nurses are not available to undertake their specified tasks. In these situations it can be useful to have a protocol in place so that another person can take over, while still maintaining the same standard of care.

What is a protocol?

A protocol is a defined method of completing a task that is usually written down for reference: for example, a practice protocol for triaging patients. A protocol will only work if it is known to exist, is displayed or kept in an area that is easily accessible to all members of staff who may require it, and has been seen by everyone before it is required. Protocols can also be used as a revision guide or a learning aid for newly employed personnel.

Why have protocols?

Protocols are very useful for inexperienced staff to refer to, especially when the consulting nurse is off duty or on holiday. A fellow member of staff can refer to the diabetic clinic protocol, for example, to know what to include in the clinic.

In practice, veterinary nurses follow policies and protocols all the time. Most of them are not written down, but you all know them – for instance, at what age does the veterinary practice recommend neutering in dogs and cats? How would you proceed to book that animal in for the procedure? Are you only permitted to book in a specified number of procedures per day and for specified veterinary surgeons?

Recognising a potential need for a protocol

If you are asked the same question over and over again about what to do in a certain situation, this may be an area where a written protocol would be useful. Staff members can then refer to the written (or online) version, without having to ask the specific veterinary nurse repeatedly.

If you ever think 'What would happen if I wasn't here?', you have identified the need for a protocol that other members of staff can refer to. It is important for the consulting nurse to have these protocols in place, as the same nurse cannot be on duty all the time.

Writing the protocol

In order to write the protocol correctly, all relevant information on the subject needs to be gathered. Some questions you need to be ask are:

- What is the ultimate goal for this protocol?
- Are there different options/routes to follow, depending on the situation?
- What if something doesn't work?
- How often should the protocol be reviewed?

The protocol has to be based on the answers to these question, and the practice's policies. Input from a veterinary surgeon with an interest in the particular subject, who can review what has been written, is essential. If any staff member has a particular interest in a topic, ask them to help draft a protocol or review what you have written. Involving other colleagues will increase the likelihood of the protocol being followed.

A protocol does not have to be just a list of instructions; it could be a table, or a photocopy of something really useful from a book, which you think may be helpful in practice. The completed protocol should be copied to all relevant personnel. It should then be made accessible to anyone who may need to refer to it, either as hard copy or online.

Reviewing protocols

All protocols need to be checked regularly, and rewritten if necessary. Like anything in veterinary medicine, protocols can be superseded by new information, products and procedures. Always be welcoming to new ideas from colleagues who may know of an easier, more effective way of performing a particular task than the existing protocol requires.

If the initial version of the protocol does not work, is it easy to fix? Can the protocol be amended to deal with the problem that arose?

The use of protocols can aid in clinical decisions and nursing regimes for certain medical conditions. For student nurses or inexperienced staff members, protocols can be extremely useful if used correctly and kept updated.

Part II

Nutrition and Diet

7 Food and Feeding

In order to recommend a diet or give general advice about diets it is important to be able to understand the packaging and labelling of diets, feeding techniques, and how to calculate the energy requirements and thus the feeding quantities of diets. Many owners will ask if a specific diet that they are currently feeding is any good for their pet. In these cases it is just not the food that needs to be looked at but also the pet's overall body condition, energy levels and health status. A diet may suit one dog exceptionally well and another not so well. Other factors such as availability of the diet, pack sizes that the diet is sold in, price and owner preferences also need to be taken into account. Owner preferences can include whether the food is 'ethically' manufactured or organic, wet rather than dry foods, or even the avoidance of diets that contain artificial colorants and preservatives.

Labelling of diets

In order to correctly identify the diet of choice for an individual animal, the diet needs to be evaluated. This is achieved by analysis of the ingredients. The labelling of pet foods, whether life stage diets or prescription diets, must contain several items of information (Figure 7.1).

Diets that are fed for a clinical application are required to show further information relating to the particular purpose the diet is designed for and the species being fed. The type and levels of nutrients, additives and characteristics of the diet that have been modified to suit this purpose should be stated. Also stated is the length of time during which the animal should be fed the diet – this is normally 6 months. Many diets can be fed for longer than this, but it is recommended that all patients on clinical diets on a long-term basis should have a medical examination at least every 6 months. For example, cats on diets designed to prevent feline lower urinary tract disease (FLUTD) should have a urine sample analysed a minimum of every 6 months or, for renal patients, should have repeated blood biochemistry and haematological analysis.

The Consulting Veterinary Nurse, First Edition. Nicola Ackerman.
© 2012 John Wiley & Sons, Ltd. Published 2012 by John Wiley & Sons, Ltd.

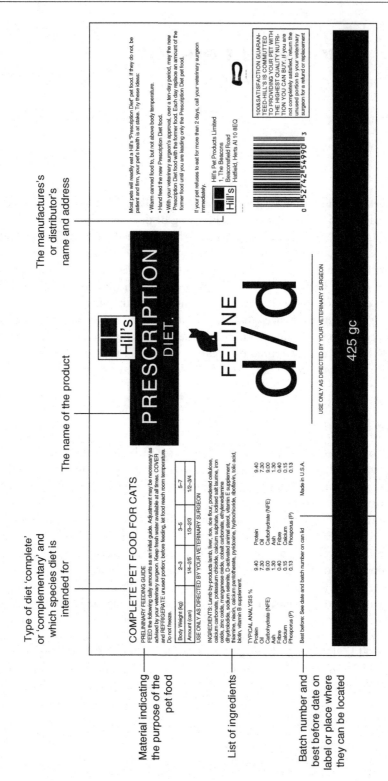

Type of diet 'complete' or 'complementary' and which species diet is intended for

The name of the product

The manufactures's or distributor's name and address

Material indicating the purpose of the pet food

List of ingredients

Batch number and best before date on label or place where they can be located

Figure 7.1 Example of a pet food label, demonstrating the legally required information that must be included. Reproduced with permission from Hill's Pet Nutrition, Inc.

Table 7.1 Comparison between dry and moist diets when calculated on a dry matter basis (DMB)

Food A	Food B
75% moisture, 10% protein Amount of dry matter (100 − 75) = 25% Protein content = 10/25 × 100 = 40%	20% moisture, 10% protein Amount of dry matter (100 − 20) = 80% Protein content = 10/80 × 100 = 12.5%
Thus Food A contains over three times as much protein as Food B on a DMB	

Comparison of foods

The quality of the food cannot be assessed from the food label, especially the true digestibility of individual nutrients and the overall digestibility of the diet. The bioavailability of nutrients is not disclosed on the label, but it does need to be conveyed to owners when they compare foods. The typical analysis states the percentage of protein, oil (fat), fibre, ash and moisture (when over 14%). In the USA a guaranteed analysis is used, where percentages again are used, but a minimum and maximal value of each nutrient is given.

The moisture content of the diet has a direct effect on the remaining ingredients. Moist diets are more dilute than dry diets, so direct comparison of the typical analysis is inaccurate when moisture contents differ (Table 7.1). Comparisons should only be made on dry matter basis (DMB) percentages, or on the basis of energy content (e.g. per 100 kcal).

Proximal analysis of food

The most common method of determining the nutrient content of the diet is through proximal analysis. This method calculates the percentage of water (moisture), protein, fat, ash and crude fibre in the diet. The percentage that is left (i.e. 100% - % moisture - % crude protein - % fat - % crude fibre - % ash) is carbohydrates or nitrogen-free extract (NFE). Crude protein levels are calculated on the basis that the protein contains 16 ± 2% nitrogen. The crude protein therefore equals nitrogen × 6.25, or nitrogen divided by 0.16. Errors can occur when non-protein nitrogen compounds such as urea or ammonia are used with the product. Figure 7.2 demonstrates proximate analysis of foods.

Types of proprietary diets

Proprietary diets are those that are commercially made, i.e. processed. They fall into two basic categories – complete or complementary.

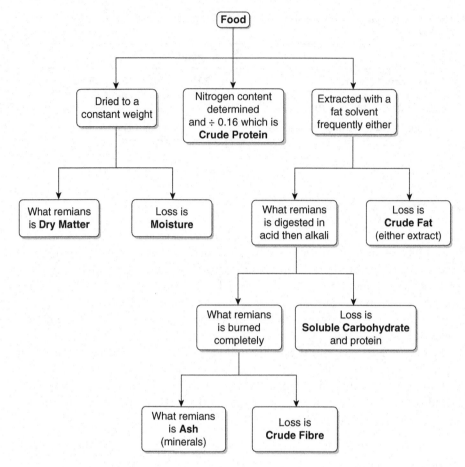

Figure 7.2   Proximate analysis of foods.

Complete diets

Complete diets provide a nutritionally balanced and adequate diet when fed as the sole source of food. All of the nutrient components are provided in the correct ratio, for the specific life stage, and do not require any additions from any another food source. In fact, adding other food sources to the diet in large quantities can make the overall daily intake of food nutritionally unbalanced.

Complementary diets

Complementary diets do not provide a nutritionally balanced diet when fed alone. These diets are designed to be fed in combination with other foods, in order to form a balanced and adequate diet. All treats and snacks are labelled as complementary foods, and thus should only make up a small portion of the daily ration.

Homemade diets

It is still relatively common for cats and dogs to be fed homemade diets. If prepared well, and with careful consideration to ensure that it is balanced, a homemade diet can serve some purpose in certain cases, e.g. in food trials. Many homemade diets contain excessive quantities of protein and carbohydrates, and are limited in vitamins and minerals, especially calcium. If owners wish to pursue the use of a homemade diet, examples of a suitable diet should be obtained from the veterinary practice. It is also advisable that the animal has its body condition score (BCS), weight and clinical health examined regularly, to ensure that the diet is balanced and no deficiencies are present. Aiding the owner in designing the diet is important, and there are simple guidelines to follow when designing a diet (Hotston-Moore 2004; see Box 7.1).

Box 7.1   Six simple guidelines to follow when designing a diet

1   Do the five main food groups appear in the diet?

- A multivitamin
- A source of minerals including trace minerals (careful consideration should be given to calcium levels)
- A fat source
- A protein source (in feline diets it is vital that an animal-sourced protein is used)
- A carbohydrate source (this also includes fibre). Sources used should be from cooked cereals, grain or potato. (Potatoes and tapioca are an excellent carbohydrate source when performing food trials, as they are not commonly used in commercial diets.)

2   What is the quality and source of the protein?

The protein levels and the protein quality within the diet are two very different things. A high protein level does not necessarily mean that the animal is receiving all of the necessary essential amino acids it requires. Skeletal muscle protein from different sources contains similar amounts of amino acids, and there is therefore no great advantage of feeding one type of meat over another, unless it is for the purpose of food trials. Novel protein sources used include duck, venison, salmon and egg. Egg is an excellent protein source (biological value 100%), and in cases where restricted protein levels are required the inclusion of egg as a protein source in the diet is highly recommended, as it ensures a high protein quality.

3   What is the fat content of the protein source?

Cuts of meat vary greatly in their content of fat. If the fat content is high other fat levels should be reduced in order to compensate for this.

4   What is the carbohydrate to protein ratio within the diet?

The carbohydrate/protein ratio should be approximately 1:1 to 2:1 for cat diets and 2:1 to 3:1 in canine diets (Hotston-Moore 2004).

(Continued)

> **5   Is there a source of vitamin and minerals?**
>
> A homemade diet will be unbalanced in terms of vitamins and minerals unless they are supplemented. When using homemade diets for food trials the use of supplements is not recommended, as this will affect the trial. As the trial is not long term, short-term deficiencies can be tolerated in many cases.
>
> **6   Is there a source of other essential nutrients?**
>
> Other essential nutrients such as essential fatty acids (EFAs), taurine and other essential amino acids (EAAs) need to be supplemented into the diet in order to ensure adequate levels. This can be achieved through the addition of oils and other supplements.

Homemade diets should be cooked, as this helps to increase the overall digestibility of the diet, and reduces the risk of food poisoning. Overcooking will result in a loss of nutrients from the diet, especially vitamins and the denaturing of proteins. There are a vast number of different homemade diets available on the internet, and they can even be designed for a specific animal and/or clinical disease.

Palatability

The palatability of a food is its degree of acceptability to an animal. Any diet must be palatable if the animal is to consume it. There are three essential components to palatability: the pet (species and individual), the environment (owner, home, lifestyle), and the food itself (smell, shape, texture, taste, nutritional composition). The first component, the pet, cannot be altered in order to enhance the palatability of the diet. The second component, the environment, can be changed in some ways. The habits of the owner around feeding time, the designated areas in which the animal is normally fed, the types of bowls used, for example, can all be changed to benefit the animal. The veterinary practice should be able to be provide guidance to the client about this. The third component, the food itself, plays the largest role in palatability, and will be discussed further.

Food aroma and temperature

The temperature of the food plays a huge role in the acceptability of the diet. Cats prefer food that is near body temperature. This is a direct reflection of their natural diet in the wild. Food which is taken straight from the fridge can be less appealing, as can foods above 40 °C /104 °F (Wills 1996).

The aroma of the diet plays a significant role in the animal's acceptance of the food. Animals that have a reduced olfactory capacity, such as older animals, sick animals and those on medications that reduce their sense of smell, can show a

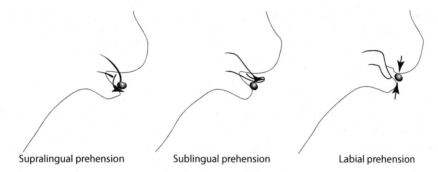

Supralingual prehension   Sublingual prehension   Labial prehension

Figure 7.3   Methods of prehension in the cat.

marked decrease in the acceptance of a diet. Cleaning any mucus from the animal's nose will help. The use of moist diets can be advantageous, as these diets give off stronger aromas.

Prehension

The way the animal picks up the food in its mouth, and the way in which it eats it, also have a role in the palatability of the diet. Cats exhibit three different methods of dry food prehension. The most common method is labial prehension. In this method the cat grasps the kibble between the incisors, without the use of the tongue. The second method, supralingual prehension, involves the cat using the dorsal side of the tongue to lap up the kibbles. The third method, sublingual prehension, occurs when the cat applies the ventral side of the tongue to the kibble, turning the kibble backwards into the mouth (Figure 7.3). Sublingual prehension is commonly used by brachycephalic breeds, such as Persians. Different kibble shapes have been shown to suit certain types of prehension; for example, almond-shaped kibbles are best suited for cats that use sublingual prehension.

In the dog, prehension does not seem to be linked to kibble shape and size, but this does affect other feeding parameters, including the time taken to eat the diet and encouraging the dog to chew the kibble rather than swallowing it whole.

Taste

Once the animal has smelt the aroma of the food, and picked it up into its mouth, taste is the third stage in food selection and an important factor that affects the palatability of the diet. Taste perception can be modulated by four factors:

- Sex: It has been found that female dogs are more receptive to sweet tastes than males. In many species pregnancy and hormonal imbalances can also affect taste and responses to taste and smells.
- Age: Taste sensitivity declines with age.
- State of health: Some diseases affect taste. These include chronic renal failure, diabetes mellitus, thyroid dysfunction and cranial trauma. Nasal discharges will also affect the ability to taste, hence the requirement to bathe nasal discharges away in order to help cats suffering from viral infections to eat.
- Drugs: For example, tetracycline alters taste perception.

The taste of the diet can be directly influenced by many factors, including the ingredients used, manufacturing practices, storage, pet food preservation systems, packaging and palatability enhancers.

Texture

The consistency of the diet has large effects on the quantity fed, the palatability (in some cases), the way in which the diet is stored and packaged, and the methods in which the animal is fed. Cats and dogs prefer meat-based canned products rather than dry expanded diets (Thorne 2005). This has been attributed to the higher moisture content, and to the fact that blood and fluids contain positive palatability factors (Thorne 2005).

Moist diets

Moist diets contain 70–85% moisture, and are extremely popular. Packaging for moist diets ranges from cans to foil trays and pouches. These diets are very palatable, and can lead to overeating and obesity. The moisture content of these diets can prove to be invaluable when you are trying to increase water content of the animal's diet, especially in cases of FLUTD. It is recommended that all cats have a portion of their diet made up of moist foods.

Semi-moist diets

Semi-moist diets contain around 30% moisture. During manufacture, the ingredients are cooked and formed into a paste which is then passed through an extruder and shaped into pieces. Acid preservatives are then added in order to inhibit bacterial and fungal growth. Corn syrup may be used to coat the pieces to prevent drying out, and to remove the availability of the moisture for bacterial and fungal growth. The syrup coating makes the pieces very palatable, but totally unsuitable for diabetic patients. Semi-moist diets should not be fed to cats as they may contain propylene glycol. Propylene glycol is an approved food additive for dog food,

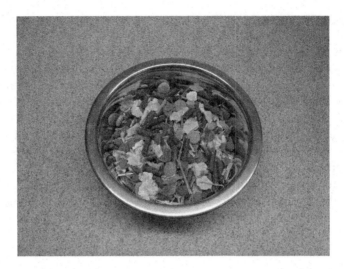

Figure 7.4 Meal-type diets.

under the category of animal feed; it is generally recognised as safe for dogs, and it is an approved food additive for human food as well. The exception is that it is prohibited for use in food for cats.

Dry diets

Dry diets contain 10–14% moisture, and can be made by a number of different methods. Using a mixture of dry flaked and crushed cereals and vegetables creates **meal-type diets** (Figure 7.4). These diets can be beneficial when catering for large numbers of animals, as each individual animal's requirements can be met; this is a common method for feeding horses. Forming the ingredients into a paste and cooking them creates **extruded diets**. This process involves steam and pressure-cooking. The cooking process can improve the digestibility of the diet, as some nutrients are broken down in the process. The extruded kibbles can then be coated in flavourings, dried and packaged.

Extruded diets tend to be complete and balanced for the life stage that they are designed for. In some species extruded and pelleted diets are preferred as they prevent selective feeding, a common problem in meal-type diets, especially in rabbits and small rodents. Extruded diets increase chewing compared to pelleted diets, thus increasing palatability, and increasing positive eating behaviour – no gulping, for example. This eating behaviour also causes an increase in the production of saliva. Extruded diets are ideal for working/performance diets, for any species, as higher fat levels can be incorporated.

Some food manufactures use a combination of extruded kibbles alongside semi-moist kibbles, as the semi-moist kibbles can aid in increasing the overall palatability of the diet.

Post-ingestion effects

Once food is consumed, the gastrointestinal tract provides many signals related to food ingestion. Distension of the stomach with food stimulates stretch and chemoreceptors. These receptors send vagal signals to the satiety centre in the brain. Both positive and negative feedback mechanisms are responsible for regulating food intake. Negative feedback mechanisms such as insulin, serotonin, leptin, neurotensin and glucagons appear to attenuate food intake. Daily administration of leptin has been shown to decrease food consumption, and thus induce weight loss (Buffington et al. 2004). Positive feedback mechanisms include the activation of the autonomic system during eating. Opioid and dopaminergic neurons are involved in the stimulation of food intake, and aid in the positive reinforcement of food intake.

Energy calculations

To ensure that the patient is receiving sufficient calories, calculations based on weight can be performed. Using the calculated energy requirement divided by the calorific value of the diet on an 'as fed' basis will result in the quantity of diet to be fed. Daily weighing of the animal and the use of BCS will confirm whether the calories provided to the animal are sufficient, adequate or excessive.

- **Basal energy requirement (BER):** The amount of energy required by a healthy animal in a thermoneutral environment, while awake but not exercising, 12 hours after eating.
- **Resting energy requirement (RER):** The RER differs from the BER as it includes energy expended for recovery from physical activity and feeding. The RER for dogs and cats is dependent on the body weight of the animal BwT and can be calculated from the following equations:

$$RER \ (kcal/day) = 70 \times BwT^{0.75} \ (if \ BwT \ is \ less \ than \ 2 \ kg)$$

or

$$30 \times (70 \times Bwt)(if \ Bwt \ is \ between \ 2 \ and \ 45 \ kg).$$

It has been calculated that RER may be 1.25 × BER, but in many texts often regard the two as interchangeable values.
- **Maintenance energy requirement (MER):** The energy required for a moderately active adult in a thermoneutral environment. This includes energy for obtaining, digesting and absorbing food in animals to maintain an optimal body weight. Average values for a dog are 2 × RER, and for cats 1.4 × RER.
- **Daily energy requirement (DER):** This represents the average daily energy requirement for any animal, dependent on life stage and activity. The DER is calculated from the RER and a life stage factor (see Box 7.2).

Box 7.2   Daily energy requirements

Cats

- Kitten (growth): 2.5 × RER
- Neutered cat: 1.2 × RER
- Entire cat: 1.4 × RER
- Active cat: 1.6 × RER
- Pregnancy: 1.6–2 × RER
- Lactation: 2–6 × RER (dependent on number of nursing kittens)

Some food manufacturers market different types of foods for neutered males and neutered female cats. There is a metabolic difference between the two sexes, but it is marginal.

Dogs

- Neutered dog: 1.6 × RER
- Entire dog: 1.8 × RER
- Active/working: 3–8 × RER
- Pregnancy (>21 days): 3 × RER
- Lactation: 4–8 × RER (dependent on number of nursing puppies)

All calculations are a rough estimate, and should be adapted to the individual depending on BCS and weight gains and losses. Illness factors have limited use in energy calculations, and nutritional assessment of the patient should be used in order to increase or decrease the amount fed.

Energy metabolism

The route by which energy is obtained from the diet is dependent on the nutrients absorbed. Figure 7.5 demonstrates the main metabolic pathways utilised in the conversion of food to energy.

The amount of energy from the diet that is ultimately available to the body is dependent on the digestibility of the diet, the amount of energy lost in urine and faeces, and the energy required to absorb the nutrients. The gross energy (GE) of the diet is the total heat produced by burning the food in a bomb calorimeter. From the GE and removing energies lost through incremental losses it is possible to calculate the net energy (NE) that can be used by the animal.

Frequently asked questions

Diet and dietary changes

Can I feed my pet a raw meat and bone diet?

There is a common trend towards feeding dogs in this manner, in order to mirror what an undomesticated dog would consume in the wild. Raw meat and bones

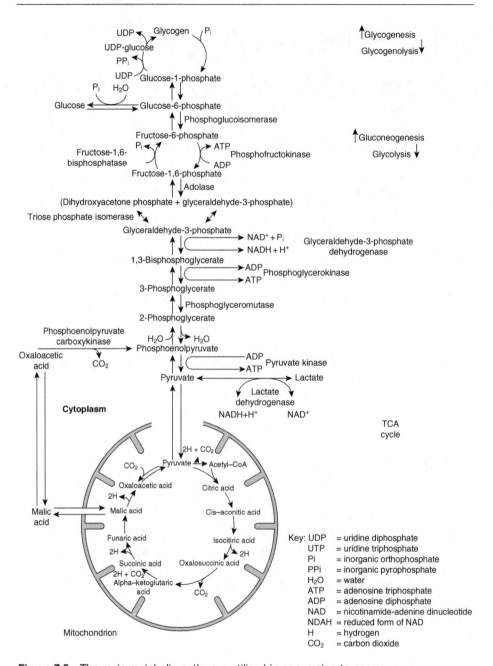

Figure 7.5 The main metabolic pathways utilised in conversion to energy.

are not an accurate reflection of a wild dog's diet, as dogs scavenge, and also consume the skin, hair and other soft tissues of their prey. Bones can also be detrimental to gastrointestinal health, and uncooked meats can contain harmful bacteria. The domesticated dogs of today have lost some of their natural immunity, and this kind of diet can therefore give them gastrointestinal upsets.

Why does my animal have diarrhoea when it changes diet?

Sudden changes in diet can cause transient diarrhoea. This can be due to the microbial population in the gastrointestinal tract having to adapt to the different nutrient make-up of the new diet. Any dietary changes should be slow, so that the microbial populations can adapt over a period of time in order to accommodate the changes. The metabolic physiology of the gastrointestinal tract also has time to adapt to the new nutrient.

How do I get my pet to change its diet?

Some animals will not want to consume a new diet, no matter how slowly you perform a transitional change. In some cases changing to an intermediate diet can help. For example, instead of changing directly on to a very restricted salt diet, you can change initially to a slightly less restricted salt diet as an intermediate step. Adding a very highly palatable diet to the new diet, and then slowly reducing this once the animal has accepted the new diet can also help. When the texture of the diet is changed, transition can be very difficult. Animals are extremely adept at eating around the desired kibble, and picking out only the bits that they want. In some exceptionally difficult cases, the use of a blender has proved very useful. The animal is then unable to pick out the bits it want, and has to consume the whole mixture. Altering the percentages of old and new diet will encourage the animal to move on to the new diet, and accustom it to the new taste. Once this has been achieved, blending the food less and less will increase the particle sizes until the animal is eating the diet as it comes out of the packaging.

Which diet do you recommend?

This is a very common question. To make a recommendation you must wholly support it, and be able to tell the owner why. In some circumstances some owners may not be able to afford what you recommend, or the animal may not like the diet. In these cases it can be useful to have an A list and a B list. The A list contains first-choice recommendations and premium diets. The B list tends to contain second-choice diets and possibly supermarket diets.

Food and exercising

Why does my dog or horse always defecate when exercising?

Moderate exercising and movement encourages defecation, by increasing peristalsis. This is one reason why movement is encouraged in horses with colic, and in rabbits with ileus. When exercise is intense the blood supply to the digestive system is reduced, hence the recommendation not to exercise after a meal. When an animal is extremely excited or fearful, some hormones such as adrenaline can increase the gastrointestinal emptying time. It can be completely normal for some dogs to defecate frequently during exercise. The stools normally start firm, becoming softer as the exercise increases, even passing diarrhoea. Some success in reducing the amount stools passed can achieved by feeding a low-residue diet, and by changing exercise and feeding routines. In some dogs this will not make any difference in the frequency of defecation. Reducing the excitability of the dog will make a difference, and this can only be achieved through desensitisation of the dog to excitable situations.

How long should I leave the animal after feeding before exercising?

This does depend heavily on the nutrient content of the diet. High-fat diets will take longer to leave the stomach than carbohydrate diets. It is recommended that at least 1 hour be left before exercising.

Is there any truth in the idea that you should withhold food and large amounts of water after exercising?

The consumption of large amounts of food and water after exercising should be avoided, until the animal's body has returned to its resting status. Water can be offered, but in small quantities.

References

Buffington CAT, Holloway C, Abood SK. *Manual of Veterinary Dietetics*. St Louis, MO: Elsevier Saunders, 2004.

Hotston-Moore P. *Fluid Therapy for Veterinary Nurses and Technicians*. Edinburgh: Butterworth Heinemann, 2004.

Thorne J. To supplement or not to supplement? Part 1. *VN Times* 2005; Dec:10–11.

Wills JM. Basic Principles of nutrition and feeding. In: Kelly N, Wills JM, eds. *Manual of Companion Animal Nutrition and Feeding*. Gloucester: BSAVA Publications, 1996, pp. 10–21.

Suggested further reading

Agar S. *Small Animal Nutrition*. Edinburgh: Butterworth Heinemann, 2001.

8 Feeding Behaviours

Finicky feeding behaviour

Fastidious or finicky eating behaviours can make a transition to a new therapeutic veterinary diet almost impossible. This kind of eating behaviour is common, and can be a human-caused problem, resulting from the animal's conditioned expectations for frequent changes in the food variety or flavour. Owners will often describe their pets as a finicky eaters if they are considered to be intermittent or slow eaters. This may, however, be due to the animal being overfed, or to the animal's own autoregulation of food consumption. Assessment of the animal's body condition score (BCS) will show whether or not the animal is consuming sufficient nutrients.

Behavioural modification of the animal to counteract this feeding behaviour is difficult, as it is reliant on the owner, who is often the cause of the initial problem. Restricting the excessive rotation of different brands and flavours to less frequent changes may help resolve the problem. A ritualised feeding routine will need to be instituted: set meals at a certain time and place, with a certain brand of food. Some animals that do self-regulate may benefit from *ad libitum* feeding. This tends to be the case with small breed dogs, as owners may overestimate the amount of diet that the dog can consume at any one time. With *ad libitum* feeding it is important that the overall daily amount of diet supplied to the pet is still weighed out, and that overconsumption of calories does not occur.

Animals that have been fed a high-quality, very palatable diet on an *ad libitum* basis (mainly cats), will expect this unlimited food availability. In order to change the animal's diet, it must be made to become dependent on the owner for food. In order to accomplish this, the animal should be offered *ad libitum* feeding for two set hours per day. Once this routine has been established, the old diet should be restricted to 75% of the previous food intake, and the rest of the daily requirement made up with the new diet, placed in a separate bowl next to the old diet.

The Consulting Veterinary Nurse, First Edition. Nicola Ackerman.
© 2012 John Wiley & Sons, Ltd. Published 2012 by John Wiley & Sons, Ltd.

Food addictions

Food addictions are fairly common: one example is cats becoming addicted to tinned tuna. Addictions can lead to nutritional deficiencies, or even toxic syndromes. Counter-conditioning behavioural modifications are required over a period of time. This modification can be done by adding a distasteful substance to the food the animal is addicted to, while providing a balanced complete diet of the same flavour as the addicted food.

Food labels should be scrutinised carefully, as foods that are 'flavoured' are different from those that contain that specific food ingredient. A prime example is that 'tuna-flavoured' cat foods do not necessarily contain tuna.

Food aversions

The implications of food aversion are dramatically underestimated in veterinary practice. It is usually not advisable to institute dietary changes while clinically ill patients are hospitalised. Diets should be introduced in the home environment once the pet is more stable.

Prevention of malnutrition by ensuring adequate nutrient intake is crucial in the management of all medical and surgical cases. The veterinary nurse or technician plays a vital role in practical measures to improve adequate intake. These practical measures include the following.

History taking

Talking to the owner is invaluable. Obtaining information on preferred types and consistency of food, and the animal's eating habits, will help to getting the animal to eat. Cats can be exceptionally fastidious about the size, shape and type of bowl or saucer that they eat out of. Wide-rimmed bowls tend to be preferred, so that they have room for their whiskers.

Removal of the clinical problem

Many medical problems, e.g. renal dysfunction, can result in changes of appetite and olfaction. Pain associated with dental disease or neoplasia in the mouth will also decrease appetite. Removal of pain or the causal agent will greatly improve the well-being of the patient.

Odorous foods

Warming up the diet to body temperature can make it more appetising to the animal. Increasing the temperature will also increase the odour of the food. Use of highly odorous foods such as pilchards can help to stimulate eating. None of these measures will work, however, if the animal is unable to smell the food. Any nasal discharges need to be cleaned away before the food is offered.

Positive reinforcements

Positive reinforcements such as hand feeding can be used to promote eating. Improving the animal's general well-being, e.g. by grooming, can also aid in this process. Trying to encourage eating outside the practice environment can prove to be useful. Taking small quantities of food when exercising the animal outside, or feeding in a room away from all other animals, might encourage the animal to eat. Timid animals can benefit from having somewhere to hide away.

Food aversions can be reinforced by repeatedly offering a diet that the animal keeps refusing. Force-feeding can be used to aid encouragement to eat, but if the animal becomes distressed this can cause a negative reinforcement to eat that particular food. Any offered food that is not consumed should be removed from the animal's environment after 15 minutes. Littering the animal's cage with a carpet of different foods will not encourage it to eat.

Feeding methods

The way in which an animal consumes its diet has an impact on many different elements of its life. There are three basic methods of feeding cats and dogs: free choice (*ad libitum*), time limited or food limited. All have their advantages and disadvantages, and will suit different animals on an individual basis. Significant breed differences have been noted in the feeding behaviours of dogs: beagles and very small breed dogs have similar feeding patterns to cats, whereas poodles are said to eat only during the daylight hours. There are, however, always individuals that are exceptions.

Free choice feeding

This method of feeding tends to suit animals that will eat only what is required to meet their energy requirements. Overconsumption can lead to obesity, and in growing dogs of large and giant breeds it can also predispose to developmental orthopaedic disorders (DOD). Other disadvantages include food wastage, especially if feeding a moist diet, and competition from other animals in the environment, which can lead to overeating in some animals and consequently undereating in others. Advantages include a more constant blood level of nutrients and hormones, and a decrease in coprophagy.

Timid animals are more likely to eat if there is a longer period of access to the food, during which other animals are not present. Many of these animals tend to carry kibbles to a different site, away from the main bowl of food, and then consume them there, rather than eating in front of other animals. This method of feeding is advised with animals with or predisposed to FLUTD, because of the postprandial alkaline tide (see Chapter 33 for more details).

With a free choice diet it is still important to monitor the amount of diet consumed within a 24 hour period in order to prevent overeating.

Time-restricted meal feeding

In this method the animal is allowed free access to the food for a set period of time each day. This is usually 10–15 minutes, once or twice daily. This can be a disadvantage in small dogs, puppies and kittens: because of their limited stomach size, they do not eat sufficient food in this short time to meet their nutritional requirements.

Overconsumption can easily occur when using this feeding method, if the animal is greedy. In these cases reducing the amount of time that the animal has access to the diet, or feeding a diet of a lower energy density, is required.

Advantages of this method include aiding in house-training in puppies. A routine of feeding a puppy and then taking it outdoors can enforce house-training by taking advantage of the gastrocolic reflex.

Food-restricted meal feeding

This method requires either calculating the DER of the animal, and thus the quantity of diet that needs to be fed, or following the manufacturer's recommendations on the food packaging. The calculated DER is then divided by the energy density of the diet in order to obtain the quantity of food that should be fed.

The advantage of this method is that, when a complete balanced diet is used, you know the animal is receiving the correct amount of nutrients. This method of feeding is recommended for animals predisposed to DODs.

The disadvantage is that all animals are individuals; some have a higher metabolism or workload and require more calories. In these cases the quantities fed should be reassessed: a performance diet could be beneficial. Likewise, some animals may gain weight using this method, and in these cases a light diet could be recommended.

Suggested further reading

Bourgeois H, Elliott D, Marniquet P, et al. The influence of food characteristics on palatability. *Focus Special Edition: Dietary preferences of dogs and cats* 2004, pp. 23–36.

LeBel C, Bourdeau A, Lau D, Hunt P. Biological response to peripheral and central administration of recombinant human leptin in dogs. *Obesity Res* 1999; 7: 577–585.

Morris JG, Rogers QR, Fascettis AJ. Nutrition of healthy dogs and cats in various stages of adult life. In: Hand MS, Thatcher CD, Remillard RL, Roudebush P, eds. *Small Animal Clinical Nutrition*, 4th edition. Topkea, KS: Mark Morris Institute, 2000, pp. 529–562.

Tefend M, Berryhill SA. Companion animal clinical nutrition. In: McCurnin DM, Bassert JM, eds. *Clinical Textbook for Veterinary Technicians*, 6th edition. St Louis, MO: Elsevier Saunders, 2006, pp. 438–492.

9 Nutrition for Puppies and Kittens

Prenatal period

Gestation and lactation

Recommendations state that the bitch or queen needs to be in good condition before breeding. This includes nutritional status, up-to-date vaccinations, and any parasiticide agents administered as necessary (endo- and exo-parasiticides). It is vital that the products used are licensed for pregnant animals. A good body condition score (BCS) and muscle condition score (MCS) are also required. Bitches and queens that are overweight are more likely to present with dystocia during parturition than animals with an ideal BCS. As demonstrated in humans, obesity can also affect fertility.

During the first 6 weeks of pregnancy it is possible to maintain bitches on their original adult diet, provided that the diet is of a good quality and is not lacking in any specific nutrients. During the final trimester the bitch will require to be switched to a growth/puppy diet. Large breed puppy diets are not recommended even for large breed bitches, which will require a puppy growth diet intended for dogs under 25 kg. Large breed puppy diets have a decreased level of energy, whereas the bitch in the last 3 weeks of pregnancy especially requires energy. The bitch's weight should increase to approximately 25% more than her weight at time of breeding, although this does depend on the number in the litter. During this stage more frequent feeding maybe required owing to a decrease in the quantity of diet consumed at each meal. If the bitch is having difficulties consuming adequate calories, *ad libitum* feeding should be introduced. Fresh water must be made available at all times.

The feeding of queens during pregnancy differs from that of bitches. Queens increase food intake soon after conception, and this increases with the duration of gestation. During the first third of pregnancy the queen will lay down fat reserves, which will be used towards the end of gestation and during lactation. (Dzanis 1995).

Lactation places huge stresses on the nutritional demands of the bitch or queen. The nutritional demands can increase from 3–6 times that of maintenance, depend-

The Consulting Veterinary Nurse, First Edition. Nicola Ackerman.
© 2012 John Wiley & Sons, Ltd. Published 2012 by John Wiley & Sons, Ltd.

ing on the number in the litter. The growth diet still needs to be fed free choice (*ad libitum*). Large volumes of water will be required and must be available at all times. Peak lactation demands will occur when the litter is 3–6 weeks of age, and further nutritional support of the bitch and queen will be required then. Colostrum is vitally important to all mammals; it contains many antibodies from the mother, aiding in early immunological status of the puppies or kittens. Queens and bitches sustain a loss of body weight during lactation. *Ad libitum* feeding during pregnancy will allow for the increase in body tissue that will be metabolised during lactation and by fetal energy demands (Furniss 2006). The weaning body weight of the queen or bitch should not be less than the body weight at conception.

A worming regime for the bitch or queen and for the litter must be implemented, and will have a large effect on the nutritional status and well-being of all. The bitch needs to be wormed before breeding and from day 42 of gestation daily until 2 days after parturition. This is due to transmission of the parasite *Toxocara canis*, transplacentally and transmammarily. In the queen worming is only required after parturition as *Toxocara cati* is only transmitted transmammarily. Studies have shown that a good worming regime will result in larger, healthier puppies and kittens. The offspring will require worming depending on the dosing licence of the pharmaceutical used.

Many owners are breeding their pet for the first time, due to mismating, and having the opportunity to talk through the details of pregnancy and whelping with a veterinary professional can be very reassuring. The use of good handouts and sources of accurate information for the owner can be invaluable. Many practices put information regarding breeding and pregnancy on their own websites.

In many cases the requirement for a caesarean is the first time that the practice may be aware that the bitch was pregnant (Figure 9.1). The discharge appointment is a really good opportunity to discuss matters regarding worming, nutrition, weaning, etc. with the owner if this information is required.

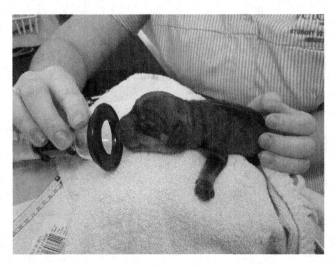

Figure 9.1   Puppy receiving oxygen post caesarean.

Postnatal period

When nursing, puppies and kittens should be vigorous and active. For the first 3–4 weeks with puppies, and 4 weeks with kittens, exclusive feeding from the mother is possible if she is healthy and well nourished. The expected weight gain of kittens should be 10–15 g/day, and puppies 2–4 g/day per kilogram of anticipated adult weight (or at least 10% gain per day) (Furniss 2006). Puppies and kittens which are not receiving sufficient milk will cry, become restless or extreme in activity and fail to achieve the expected weight gain. It should be remembered that littermates will differ, and gain weight at different rates. The veterinary nurse should recommend the owner to weigh the puppies/kittens daily.

Hand-rearing of puppies and kittens

The most obvious alternative to being reared by the mother is the use of a foster mother. If this is not possible, hand-rearing is the other alternative. Many puppy and kitten formulas are available (Figure 9.2), and each has its own feeding guidelines. The calorific needs for most nursing-age puppies and kittens is 22 to 26 kcal per 100 g body weight (Furniss 2006). The number of daily feedings is dependent on the formula guidelines, and the formula should be warmed to 37.8 °C (100 °F) before each feeding.

All equipment (bottles, teats, etc.) must be sterilised before feeding. It is usually more convenient to prepare a 24 hour supply of milk, and divide this into portions required for each meal. Prepared formula must be stored in a refrigerator; any unused prepared formula should be discarded if not used with 48 hours. Chilled

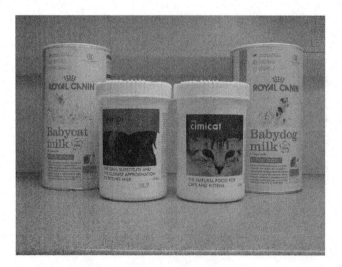

Figure 9.2 Examples of puppy and kitten formula.

prepared formula should not be fed to a puppy or kitten without warming, as this can induce colic. After feeding, the abdomen should appear enlarged but not overdistended.

Tube feeding is another method of feeding orphaned puppies or kittens. If a suckling reflex is present bottle-feeding is the preferred method, because it has fewer potential complications. When tube feeding, the formula should be warmed, and administered over a 2 minute period. This will allow sufficient time for slow filling of the stomach.

After feeding, stimulation of the anogenital area is required. This is normally done with warm, moist cotton wool and provokes the reflexes of micturition and defecation. By 3 weeks of age puppies and kittens are usually able to relieve themselves without simulated stimulation.

Weaning

The idea of solid foods can be introduced to the puppies or kittens at 3–4 weeks of age. A mixture of the mother's diet (providing it is an adequate one) mixed with warm water is ideal. At this age the puppies and kittens will show an interest and taste the food, but will not consume enough to meet nutritional requirements. Observing the mother eating the diet is important, and will encourage the puppies or kittens to start lapping. When eating their first solid food kittens do not choose the most palatable food according to innate criteria. They will choose what their mothers eat, even if their food is unusual (Wyrwicka 1978). Complete weaning can start at 6 weeks of age, and be achieved by 8 weeks. In most cases the bitch or queen will wish to spend less time nursing, and may start to get annoyed or frustrated at the youngsters when they try to suckle.

On weaning, puppies and kittens need to be fed a good-quality complete growth diet. Many breeders have different feeding programmes involving Weetabix, goat's milk, scrambled eggs, mincemeat and calcium supplements. Advising new puppy owners on a correct diet is vital. Questions should be asked about diet when the new puppy or kitten is initially presented at the veterinary practice. Most breeders who use complete growth diets will rehome animals with the recommendation that the animal remains on the same diet during this transitional period. There is no reason to change the diet unless the animal is not gaining weight adequately, if the diet is not nutritionally balanced or if the animal is grossly overweight.

Vaccination period

In many practices nurses have little input during vaccinations of puppies and kittens. The introduction of the clinic nurse at this point can prove to be beneficial. The clinic nurse is able to give more quality time to the new pet owner once the health check and vaccination has been done by the veterinary surgeon.

As puppies and kittens are due worming monthly until 6 months of age, monthly clinics are an opportunity to obtain an up-to-date weight, and discuss any matters that the owner wants advice on. A recommendation from the veterinary surgeon who carries out the initial vaccinations is paramount. Many clients don't want to 'burden' the veterinary surgeon with questions that they feel are silly. Having the opportunity to speak to a veterinary nurse can prove invaluable to new pet owners in these situations.

Feeding puppies and kittens

Puppy growth diets are divided into those designed for pups that will weigh more than 25 kg when full grown, and those that will weigh less than 25 kg. This division is due to growth rates and the age at which maturity is reached. Large breeds should grow at a slower rate over a longer period of time. Diets designed for these breeds are modified to have lower energy levels, thus preventing rapid growth rates. Historically these large breed's diets were supplemented with calcium, as it was felt that extra calcium was required to support the skeletal system during the rapid growth rate. In fact extra calcium is not required, and the calcium/phosphorus ratio should be kept in the range of 1:1 to 1.5:1. If the energy content of the diet is correct rapid growth phases are prevented, and the incidence of developmental orthopaedic disorders (DOD) is reduced.

Overfeeding should be avoided in all puppies and kittens, as it can lead to obesity in later life. Slight underfeeding, which does not induce a reduction in full growth potential, will help to increase the animal's lifespan. Despite this, dense high-energy diets are required for growth because small animals have a limited stomach capacity, which limits the quantity of food they can consume at each meal.

Weight gain needs to be assessed daily for the first few weeks of life. Once weaned and rehomed, puppies (normally at 6–8 weeks) and kittens (8–10 weeks) should be weighed at least fortnightly until 3 months old, and then monthly until 6 months old. This conveniently fits in with the required worming regime. The use of growth charts can be invaluable, and enables trends in weight gain to be monitored (Figure 9.3). Too slow a weight gain can reflect insufficient calories being consumed, or inadequate protein quality in the diet.

The addition of treats to the diet of puppies increases greatly during this phase of life, as socialisation and training occurs. Some of the pup's complete diet kibbles can be used for this purpose, which will prevent unbalancing of the diet, and can help stop bad feeding habits from being formed. Advice on healthy treat options and other methods of positive reinforcement, i.e. use of toys, social interaction and playing, should be relayed to the owner. The setting up of good feeding habits and behaviour occurs at this age, and puppies and kittens should be introduced to these from an early age.

Docosahexaenoic acid (DHA) has been shown to improve cognitive ability and visual acuity, and has been introduced into commercial puppy and kitten diets. As a result of these benefits, DHA has the potential to speed training, obedience and socialisation.

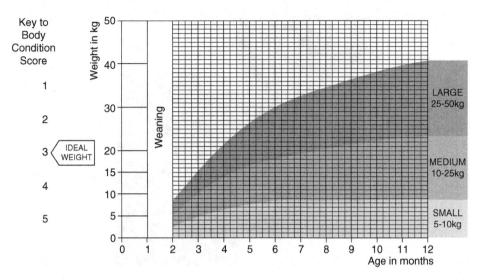

Figure 9.3   Growth charts. Reproduced with permission from Hill's Pet Nutrition, Inc.

Developmental orthopaedic disorders

The DODs are a diverse group of musculoskeletal disorders that occur in growing animals, most commonly fast-growing large- and giant-breed dogs, and horses (Richardson et al. 2000). DOD can be attributed to genetic make-up and to nutritional and stress-related aetiologies. This chapter discusses nutritionally induced aetiologies. The most commonly seen of these disorders are canine hip dysplasia (CHD) and dyschondroplasia (DCP). Osteochondrosis dissecans (OCD) is a similar condition, but occurs when inflammation is present and there is a separation between a piece of articular cartilage and the underlying bone within the joint (Figure 9.4). Other disorders coming under the umbrella of DOD include physitis (physeal dysplasia or epiphysitis), angular limb deformities and vertebral abnormalities (wobbler syndrome). The skeletal system is most susceptible to physical and metabolic insult during the first 12 months of life, due to the heightened metabolic activity. (Richardson and Toll 1996). Problems associated with dietary excesses are more likely at this stage, especially in dogs fed a high-quality growth food that is further supplemented with minerals, vitamins and energy (Kallfelz and Dzanis 1989). Lesions can appear in physeal or articular cartilage as disturbances of endochondral ossification (Daemmrich 1991).

Nutritional aims for animals predisposed to DODs include:

- Feed a complete and balanced diet that does not precipitate any predisposition to DODs
- When DODs do occur, the diet needs to limit any further damage that could be induced through poor or inadequate nutrition

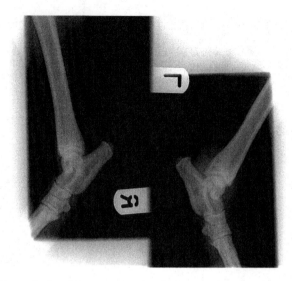

Figure 9.4 Radiograph showing osteochondrosis dissecans, a developmental orthopaedic disorder.

Clinical nutrition

Fat

Excessive dietary energy intake may support a growth rate that is too fast for correct skeletal development. Dietary fat is the primary contributor to excess energy intake (Richardson and Toll 1996), because fats have twice the calorific density of proteins and carbohydrates. Fat levels should therefore be monitored in large breed diets. Excessive energy intake can easily occur in diets with higher fat levels. Dietary energy in excess of the animal's requirements will be stored as body fat. The role of BCS is therefore important, in order to monitor energy intake. Diets formulated for large and giant breeds have a decreased energy density in comparison to small and medium breed puppy diets.

Protein

Protein levels in diets aimed at fast-growing animals have higher protein levels. The proteins used should be of a high quality and easily digestible. In dogs, protein excess has not shown to negatively affect calcium metabolism or skeletal development (Richardson et al. 2000). A growth diet for dogs should contain more than 22% protein (dry matter basis) of a high biological value (Dzanis 1995).

Carbohydrates

The carbohydrate content of the diet also needs to be balanced. Levels need to be sufficient to provide adequate calories to the animal, but not high enough to encourage excess weight gain. The type of carbohydrate in the diet is important. In cats and dogs the carbohydrate content has to be of a highly digestible nature, especially in small breeds of dogs and kittens. In horses and rabbits the type of carbohydrate in the diet needs to reflect how these animals obtain calories from hindgut fermentation; this means that the carbohydrates present need to consist mainly of fibre. In kittens and small breed puppies this level of fibre would decrease the digestibility of the diet and thus they would not be able to consume the calorific quantities required for growth, because of their limited stomach size.

Vitamins and minerals

The levels of calcium in the diet is vitally important in the development of orthopaedic disorders in large breed dogs. Equally so is the ratio of calcium to phosphorus. Excessive dietary phosphorus consistently produces lesions of DCP (Dzanis 1995). An excess of calcium causing hypercalcaemia will result in excess bone deposition, which will interfere with normal bone development.

The role of vitamins A and D in causing skeletal problems has been well documented. Vitamin A is an essential factor in bone metabolism, especially osteoclastic activity. Deficiencies or excesses in vitamin A can lead to metabolic bone disease, but are fortunately rare because of the use of commercial balanced diets. Metabolites of vitamin D aid in the regulation of calcium metabolism and therefore of skeletal development. Deficiency of vitamin D (rickets) is rare, again due to the use of commercial diets. Excessive amounts of vitamin D will lead to hypercalcaemia and hyperphosphataemia; clinical signs also include anorexia, polydipsia, polyuria, muscle weakness, generalised soft tissue mineralisation and lameness (Richardson et al. 2000).

Feeding animals with DODs

Puppies

The feeding of an animal with a DOD, or predisposed, must be done on an individual basis, as growth rates and requirements differ greatly. Physical evaluation and BCS should be performed at least every 2 weeks. Care must be taken when trying to avoid developmental problems by changing from a puppy diet to an adult maintenance diet, in order to avoid excess calcium and energy levels. Maintenance foods have a lower energy density than growth diets, so the puppy must eat greater amounts of the diet to reach its energy requirements. Problems can arise if calcium levels in the two diets are similar; the puppy will end up consuming greater amounts of calcium than if fed the growth diet.

Owners should be advised that calcium supplements should not be given to growing puppies, unless prescribed by a veterinary surgeon. Owners should be made aware of the risk of DODs, and reassured that commercial growth diets contain all the required calcium needed.

If a DOD has occurred, then a review of the animal's diet and BCS is required (see box). Nutrition can be used to aid in prevention of DOD, but its role once the disease has been acquired is limited. It should always be remembered that food manufacturer's recommendations are just that: reassessment of the animal over regular periods is the best method of obtaining a feeding plan and the method by which the animal is being fed. Trauma to the joints should be minimised by limiting exercise until the clinical signs disappear (see Box 9.1).

Box 9.1   Key points for nutrition for animals with DODs

- Ensure a correct calcium/phosphorus ratio
- Feed a controlled energy level, suitable for the individual
- Regularly assess weight and BCS
- Use of a growth chart is advisable in the monitoring of growth rates

---

Junior and adolescent diets for dogs

Some commercial dog food brands offer a junior or adolescent choice of diet. The role of these diets can be beneficial in puppies that require an intermediate diet prior to moving onto an adult maintenance diet. For those brands that do not provide a large breed puppy diet, the use of this junior/adolescent diet is necessary to prevent rapid growth rates. When large breed puppy diets are being fed, changing to a junior or adolescent diet is not required as large breed puppy diets have a lower energy content than small and medium breed puppy diets.

The adult phase is defined from when maturity has been reached until physiological changes occur due to the ageing process. The age at which the adult phase starts depends mainly on breed variations. Smaller breeds can reach full maturity from 6 months, larger and giant breeds from 12–18 months. Each animal should have their diet altered to meet the its individual needs (Table 9.1). The quantity of diet fed will depend on the quality of the diet, amount of exercise the animal receives, neutering status and metabolism. Breeds that are predisposed to weight gain should have their weight, BCS and MCS monitored throughout this life phase. Changes of metabolism after neutering should be noted to owners, and use of 'light' diets or diets specifically aimed at neutered animals should be advocated. These diets are designed to prevent weight gain, not aid in weight loss.

Table 9.1   Average maintenance energy requirements for dogs at different life stages

Age (years)	kcal ME/kg bwt$^{0.75}$	kJ ME/kg bwt$^{0.75}$
1–2	132	550
3–7	115	480
>7	100	415

Frequently asked questions

Diets for puppies and kittens

Can I give my puppy or kitten milk?

Once a puppy or kitten has been weaned from its mother, there is no nutritional reason to provide milk. The use of cow's or goat's milk is not advised as it contains higher levels of lactose than bitch's or queen's milk, and can trigger food intolerances. This also includes commercially manufactured milk for cats. Some of these products even have a disclaimer on the packaging, warning of this problem.

Should I stick to breeder's dietary recommendations?

If the animal is on a good-quality, complete balanced diet that is suitable for that individual then there is no need to initiate a change. If the owner is unhappy about the diet, or the diet is not suitable, then it should be changed. Some owners worry about not wishing to continue with the breeder's recommendation, but they should also remember that the pet now belongs to them, and it is their choice.

Can I feed my puppy bones?

Any one working within the veterinary practice setting has seen the consequences of allowing dogs to eat bones – gut perforations, diarrhoea etc. Puppies' teeth are also fairly weak in comparison to those of adult dogs, and can easily break. The recommended advice to give to owners is that no bones should be fed to dogs.

How often should I feed my puppy?

Feeding schedules should be based on the individual. Some small breed puppies will have difficultly consuming more than a very small meal, due to their limited stomach size, and may therefore require more frequent meals. Frequency of feeding also depends on the age of the animal. When advising clients on their puppy's meal frequency these points should be conveyed, and a decision should be made based on the answers. Some puppies will self-limit and free choice feeding is suitable; some will benefit from 3–4 meals per day.

My large breed puppy is 8 months old and overweight. Which diet should it be on?

A full dietary history is required in these cases as excess weight could be due to too much of the diet being fed, treats, table scraps and training aids. Transferring the puppy on to an adult diet can help, but it should be remembered that the dog will need to consume more in order to have the correct energy intake, and this will mean an increase in calcium levels; excessive calcium could be consumed as a consequence. Reducing the amount of puppy food being fed and the removal of any other foods should be encouraged, alongside exercise levels.

Dietary changes

Why does my animal have diarrhoea when it changes diet?

Changes in diet can cause transient diarrhoea. This can be due to the microbial population in the gastrointestinal tract having to adapt to the different nutrient make-up of the new diet. Any dietary changes should be slow, so that the microbial populations can adapt over a period of time in order to accommodate the changes. The metabolic physiology of the gastrointestinal tract also has time to adapt to the new nutrient.

Which diet do you recommend?

This is a very common question. To make a recommendation you must wholly support it, and be able to tell the owner why. In some circumstances some owners may not be able to afford what you recommend, or the animal may not like the diet. In these cases it can be useful to have an A list and a B list. The A list contains first-choice recommendations and premium diets. The B list tends to contain second-choice diets and possibly supermarket diets. Use of 'costs per day' for feeding can show owners that a diet that is perceived as expensive can prove to be very cost effective on a day to day basis as less is fed per day.

References

Dzanis DA. The AAFCO dog and cat food nutrient profiles. *In:* Bonagura JD et al. *Current Veterinary Therapy XII.* Philadelphia: W.B. Saunders, 1995, pp. 1418–1421.

Daemmrich K. Relationship between bone growth in large and giant dogs. *J Nutr* 1991;121: 114–121.

Furniss G. Puppy and kitten nutrition. *VN Times* 2006; June:26–28.

Kallfelz FA, Dzanis DA. Overnutrition: an epidemic problem in pet animal practice? *Vet Clin North Am Small Anim Pract* 1989; 19:433–446.

Richardson DC, Toll PW. Relationship of nutrition to developmental skeletal disease in young dogs. *Vet Clin Nutr* 1996; 3(3):6–13.

Richardson DC, Zentek J, Hazewinkel HAW, et al. Developmental orthopaedic disease of dogs. *In:* Hand MS, Thatcher CD, Remillard RL. *Small Animal Clinical Nutrition*, 4th edition. Topeka, KS: Mark Morris Institute, 2000, pp. 505–528.

Wyrwicka W. Imitation of mother's inappropriate food preference in weanling kittens. *Pavlov J Biol Sci* 1978; 13(2):55–72.

10 Nutritional Assessment

Body condition scoring

There are many recommendations regarding the calculation of an individual animal's ideal or optimal weight. Recording the animal's weight and body condition score (BCS) as a puppy or kitten and throughout the growth phase allows monitoring of its body condition. Many practitioners take the animal's weight as recorded at the time of the first annual vaccination (about 1 year old) as the individual's ideal weight. This may be a true reflection, but if the animal was overfed during the growth phase this weight will be an overestimation. In larger breeds, on the other hand, maturity and full adult size will not have been reached at the age of 1 year, and the use of this weight will be an underestimation of ideal adult body weight. The use of breed guidance charts is not advised as there can be huge variations within breeds and this method does not take frame size into consideration.

When calculating an ideal body weight for an individual, the animal must be visibly assessed and palpated. Advising an owner what their animal should weigh, if it has never been seen by the practice before, is not recommended – for example, if an owner phones and asks what is the ideal weight for their terrier, which you have never seen. Use of the body condition score (BCS) index is the method of choice (Figure 10.1), but it cannot recommend an actual figure for the ideal body weight. The BCS can be based on a five-, seven-, or nine-point scale. Use of all these different methods, palpating the animal and reassessment after a period of weight gain or loss will provide the best method for calculating an ideal weight (Figure 10.2).

Some aspects of the BCS index do not suit certain breeds. For example, whippets and greyhounds in good condition have limited fat cover. A muscle condition score (MCS) should be used alongside the BCS (Figure 10.3). It is especially important to use the MCS when initiating a weight loss diet, as dramatic losses could be due to a drop in muscle mass and this needs to be prevented. Owners should be taught how to assess their own pet's BCS in order to determine adequate food intake (Figure 10.4).

The Consulting Veterinary Nurse, First Edition. Nicola Ackerman.
© 2012 John Wiley & Sons, Ltd. Published 2012 by John Wiley & Sons, Ltd.

BCS 1 Emaciated Obvious loss of muscle mass, no body fat or muscle mass. Ribs, spine, pelvic bones easily seen.	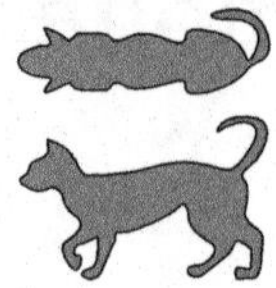	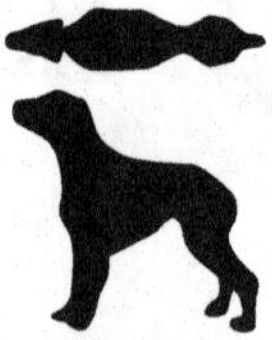
BCS 2 Thin The ribs and pelvic bones are less prominent, Waist and abdomen tuck-up when looking from the side, No palpable fat, but muscle present.	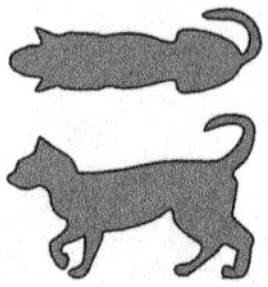	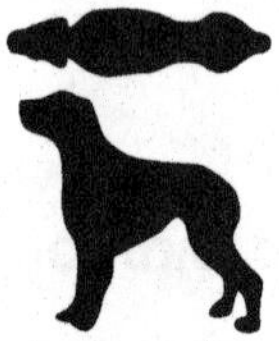
BCS 3 Moderate (Ideal) Hourglass figure less prominent (waist line), abdominal tuck present. Ribs can be felt but not seen.	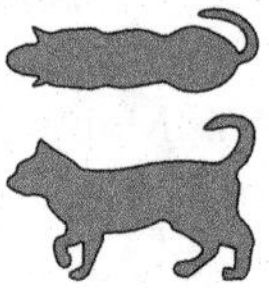	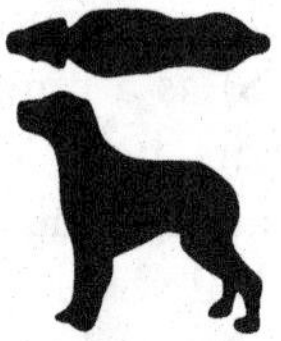
BCS 4 Overweight General fleshy appearance, waistline disappearing. Fat pads starting to form especially at base of tail.	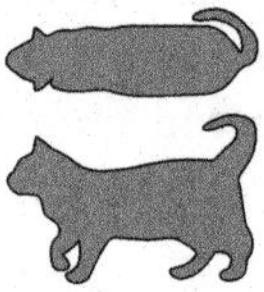	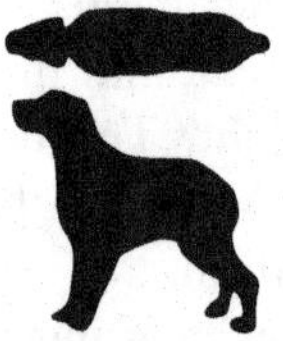
BCS 5 Obese Sagging abdomen, large fat deposits over the thorax, abdomen and pelvis, Ribs no longer palpable.	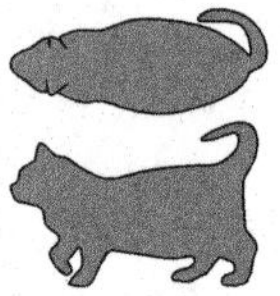	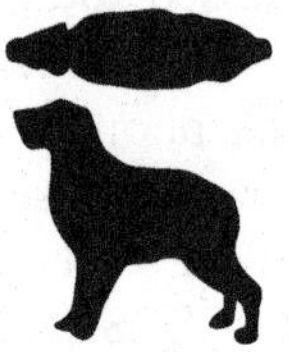

Figure 10.1 Body condition scores (five-point scale).

All of these methods are subjective, but adequate for their purpose. Other very sophisticated techniques are currently used in human patients or in research work, e.g. multiple-frequency bioelectrical impedance, dual-energy radiographic absorptiometry (DEXA) and neutron activation (Michel 2000).

'Overcoat syndrome' occurs if the animal has an MCS of 1 or 2 but is carrying excessive amounts of weight. The large fat deposits mask muscle wastage. This can easily occur in animals that suffer from a dramatic decrease in food consumption, e.g. acute anorexia. Other aspects of physical examination of the patient should be taken into consideration, including hair coat quality and skin condition,

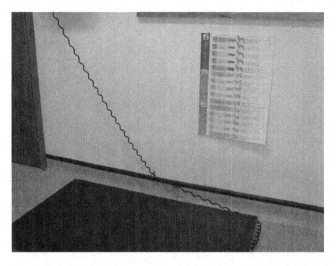

Figure 10.2   Placement of a BCS chart next to weighing scales should be encouraged.

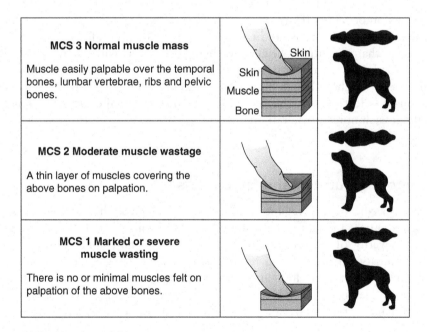

Figure 10.3   Muscle condition scores.

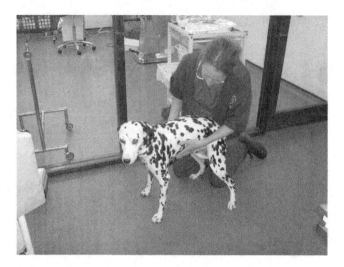

Figure 10.4 Pet owners should be taught how to BCS their own animals.

evidence of peripheral oedema or ascites (which may indicate hypoproteinemia), and clinical signs that indicate certain deficiencies in micronutrients, e.g. neck ventroflexion or tetany (Harris and Gee 2005a, 2005b).

The use of BCS can prove to be very useful for patients suffering from chronic conditions that can affect weight and body condition. Patients suffering from cardiac conditions can develop ascites, and this fluid collection can cause an overall gain in body weight although the patient's BCS may actually be decreasing as lean body mass is lost. This highlights the importance of monitoring BCS alongside weight at each nurse consultation.

Monitoring nutritional interventions

Once a specific dietary regime has been recommended, the animal should be reassessed after an appropriate period of time. This period depends on the animal, severity of disease (if any present), original nutritional status and the type of nutritional intervention received. Regular weighing of the animal, BCS, MCS and blood haematology and biochemistry parameters can all be utilised in these cases (Harris and Gee 2005a, 2005b). Animals that are placed on diets that alter urinary parameters, e.g. pH, should have these parameters monitored regularly.

References

Harris P, Gee H. Condition scoring and weight estimation: practical tools – 1. *Vet Rev* 2005a; Nov:15–18.

Harris P, Gee H. Condition scoring and weight estimation: practical tools – 2. *Vet Rev* 2005b; Dec:41–43.

Michel KE. Nutritional assessment. In: Hand MS, Thatcher CD, Remillard RL, Roudebush P, eds. *Small Animal Clinical Nutrition*, 4th edition. Topeka, KS: Mark Morris Institute, 2000, pp. 554–555.

11 Dietary Transitions

Cats and dogs

The length of the transition period of for transferring over to a new diet depends on the individual animal. Having detailed information that can be relayed to the owner is important, as an unsuccessful transition to a new diet can put the owner off the new diet completely, and may adversely affect the prospect of changing in the future.

Longer transition periods may be required when transferring from a life stage diet to a prescription diet. This is dependent on the changes in the ratio of nutrients in the diet (protein, fat, fibre levels) and/or alterations in metabolism (diarrhoea, fat maldigestion). In some cases transition to an intermediary diet may be required. An average transitional period is 3–4 days, adjusting the proportions the two diets daily. With diets that have a larger change in nutrient levels a longer transition period may be required, both for reasons of compliance and to allow time for the physiological changes in the digestive system to occur. Transition periods of up to 21–28 days are not uncommon, especially in animals that are 'fussy' with their nutritional habits.

Birds

Birds can be especially fastidious about changes of diet: patience and persistence are required. The recommended diet for companion kept birds (e.g. parrots) is a complete balanced pelleted diet. Some will immediately convert to pellets but some take longer, especially those who are 'seed junkies'. In order to wean the bird off its existing diet, a few days before attempting the changeover reduce the amount of seed that is being fed and do not top up any food that is already there. This will encourage the bird to eat all of the diet being offered, and not just pick out its favourite bits. On the day that conversion is to start, offer the bird a small amount of its normal diet (whether it is seeds or pellets) and leave this in the cage

The Consulting Veterinary Nurse, First Edition. Nicola Ackerman.
© 2012 John Wiley & Sons, Ltd. Published 2012 by John Wiley & Sons, Ltd.

for half an hour. This will ensure that the bird has received a meal. After half an hour remove this food and replace it with a small amount of the new diet; this will be left with the bird for the remainder of the day. Parrots are naturally inquisitive and will investigate the new diet. If the regular diet is left in the cage the parrot will be less likely to investigate the new diet, and to eat it. It is important to offer only a limited amount of the new diet, as larger amount will encourage the bird to play with its food and rummage looking for its regular food, especially if it cannot see the bottom of the dish. For the evening meal it is always recommended to give birds fresh fruit and vegetables (even when feeding a completed pelleted diet). If the bird will not eat fruit and vegetables, the original diet should be offered. This way you are sure that the bird has had an evening meal.

The following day repeat the same pattern, but only leave the original diet in the cage for a shorter time, approximately 20–25 minutes. Each day, reduce the amount of time that the bird has with the original diet in the morning, and increase the time it has with the new diet during the day.

Converting a bird's diet in this manner takes a lot of time and determination. Birds that are addicted to high-fat seeds can be very stubborn, but the key is to be more determined than the bird. By offering fruit and vegetables you are ensuring that the bird will not starve. In some cases, no matter how you persist in the conversion, the bird does not acknowledge the pellets as food. Methods to combat this include serving the pellets in the same way that the original diet was served, encouraging the bird to copy someone (or another bird) consuming the pellets, or moistening the pellets with the bird's favourite fruit juice.

Rabbits

Any diet changes need to be done slowly. This is even more important in rabbits than in other species because of the changes in gut flora that will need to occur in order for the animal to digest the new diet. Unduly rapid changes can lead to groups of bacteria that are no longer required dying off quickly. This causes bacterial endotoxins to be released into the gut lumen and subsequently absorbed into the bloodstream. When changes in diet are made over a period of time, the normal gut flora populations adapt slowly, without releasing high levels of endotoxins.

12 Methods of Increasing Water Consumption

The consumption of increased quantities of water is required for certain clinical diseases or disorders. Encouraging an animal to increase its water consumption can be difficult, and a number of different methods may be required in order to achieve the consumption of sufficient quantities.

Cats

Cats can be extremely fastidious in what, when and where they eat or drink. In order to increase water consumption, the availability of water needs to be increased. This can be achieved by placing more water bowls around the cat's environment (both inside and outside the house), using different types of water. Tap water, which is chlorinated, has a characteristic smell that is even more noticeable to a cat. Allowing the water to stand for a period of time removes a large proportion of the chlorine and makes it more palatable to the cat.

Cats that live in a multi-cat household can find eating and drinking alongside other cats very intimidating. Making food and water available in a place where the particular cat feels safe can be beneficial.

The water content of the diet should also be increased; this can involve changing the cat over to a moist diet, or adding water to a moist diet. Cats tend not to consume dry biscuits that have had water added to them.

Dogs

Encouraging dogs to drink more fluids can be easier in some cases than it is for cats. Again, it is important to increase the availability of water to the animal, and allow the water to stand for a period of time. The use of flavoured waters can tempt some dogs, but be careful of brands that are high in sugar. Ice cubes can also be used, and are especially useful in hot temperatures.

The Consulting Veterinary Nurse, First Edition. Nicola Ackerman.
© 2012 John Wiley & Sons, Ltd. Published 2012 by John Wiley & Sons, Ltd.

Rabbits

Encouraging a rabbit to drink more fluids is very difficult, but can be achieved. Thought should be given to the type of water container that the rabbit drinks from. Does the rabbit prefers a bowl or water bottle? The use of grasses and hays that have either been soaked or are wet can be advantageous. Spraying the grass with water before letting the rabbit out can help its increase water consumption.

Birds/reptiles

Watching these animals in the wild can demonstrate ideal ways of increasing water consumption in these species. Many birds and reptiles obtain fluids from rainfall dripping from leaves. Setting up a drip line that drips water on to foliage can actively encourage the animal to drink more. The use of rabbit/small animal water bottles has proved to be extremely useful with birds, with parrots especially liking to use this method. Water can also be injected into whole prey in order to increase water consumption.

13 Dietary Supplements

Antioxidants

The use of antioxidants in the diet is becoming more widely recognised as a positive influence in the health of animals and humans. Antioxidants are used to neutralise the ill effects of free radicals (reactive oxygen species, ROS) within the body. Free radicals are produced as by-products of chemical reaction necessary to sustain life, e.g. cellular respiration. The damage caused is dependent on the balance between the antioxidants and free radicals within the body. There are conditions that are associated with an increase in oxidative stress (see Box 13.1).

Box 13.1   Conditions associated with oxidative stress

- Ageing
- Arthritis
- Cancer
- Cardiovascular disease
- Cataracts
- Chronic pancreatitis
- Cognitive dysfunction
- Diabetes
- Haemolytic anaemia
- Infectious disease
- Liver disease
- Obesity
- Sepsis

The influence of free radical scavengers (vitamins E and C, carotenoids and selenium) is significant. Free radicals play a role in the ageing process, contributing to the development and/or exacerbation of a wide variety of degenerative diseases. There are many factors that can contribute to excessive levels of free radicals being produced. These include exposure to UV light and radiation, air pollution (including cigarette smoke), residues from herbicides and pesticides, and illness and the medications used to treat it. In human medicine, patients with some illnesses,

The Consulting Veterinary Nurse, First Edition. Nicola Ackerman.
© 2012 John Wiley & Sons, Ltd. Published 2012 by John Wiley & Sons, Ltd.

Table 13.1 Examples of some dietary supplements from plant sources, and their functions in supporting the immune function

Source	Function in aiding the immune system
Garlic	Augments macrophage and T-cell functions, inhibits tumour growth
Ginseng	Activation of a Th-1 type cellular immunity, enhances bacterial clearance, and has been shown to decrease lung pathology in rats
Grapeseed extract	Cytotoxic effect against some cancer cells, and increases the resistance against oxidative stress
Green tea	Ameliorates tumour-related immune dysfunction
Blue-green algae	Increases humoral and cell-mediated immunity. Increases immune cell translocation and activity
Echinacea	Increase antigen-specific immunoglobulin production. Enhances killer cell cytotoxicity

including diabetes mellitus, arthritis and cancers, are actively encouraged to take antioxidants.

Due to improved medical care, nutrition and veterinary guidance, animals are living longer. The incidence of cognitive dysfunction is increasing, and the use of nutrition in these cases has proved to be beneficial (see Chapter 23).

The interaction between nutrition and immune function is well documented. Any diet that it deficient in some nutrient – protein, energy, minerals, vitamins or fats – will impair immune function. Supplements or nutraceuticals that improve immune function are now available commercially. These include both antioxidants and other ingredients that are not traditionally recognised as nutritional requirements of mammals. These compounds may be derived from foods or food ingredients (e.g. garlic, grape seed extracts, green tea and isoflavones), or from herbs and botanicals (see Table 13.1) (Hayek et al. 2004).

Pre- and probiotics

Prebiotics are substances that are able to alter the gastrointestinal flora in a way that benefit the gut microorganisms. Probiotics, on the other hand, are a live microbial feed supplement, which benefits the host animal by improving the gastrointestinal microbial population. Probiotics generally used are comprised of lactic acid bacteria such as *Lactobacilli, Streptococci* and *Bifidobacteria*. Probiotics have shown to be beneficial following acute gastroenteritis or a course of antibiotics, especially in hindgut fermenters such as rabbits and horses. Live yoghurt has similar beneficial effects: the yoghurt reinforces the gastrointestinal mucosal barrier and helps stimulate gastrointestinal immunity.

Whether the bacteria can survive the acidic environment of the stomach has been questioned; hence the use of prebiotics has been stated to be more advantageous than that of probiotics. If probiotics are administered, they need to be given in large enough numbers and potentially on a daily basis. Yeasts have also been included in some probiotic preparations. Their role is to aid in improving the digestibility of fibre and other nutrients. Populations of yeasts do not seem to be maintained within the established gastrointestinal flora, and thus in order to maintain their effect, administration on a daily basis is required.

The three main mechanisms of action for probiotics are:

- **Competitive exclusion:** Colonisation sites within the gastrointestinal tract and nutrients within the gut are utilised by the probiotics. This reduces the availability of resources to the potentially pathogenic bacteria. Chronic gut dysbiosis (when undesirable microorganisms take over in large numbers) can have detrimental effects on the immune system of the digestive system (Thorne 2005).
- **Immunomodulation:** A synergistic effect exists between probiotics and the stimulation and functioning of the immune system.
- **Digestive efficiency:** Probiotic microflora have an important role in aiding the breakdown of complex food nutrients.

Prebiotics are specific nutrients that encourage the growth of beneficial bacterial population (e.g. specific types of fibre). Benefits that the host will experience from this manipulation of the gastrointestinal bacteria include:

- Inhibition of potential pathogenic bacteria, which will cause a reduction in endotoxins, carcinogens and substances associated with putrefaction
- Stimulation of gastrointestinal immunity
- Increased synthesis of vitamins, especially B complex and K
- Increased absorption of nutrients
- Improved faecal consistency
- Increased production of volatile fatty acids (VFA)/short-chain fatty acids (SCFA).

VFA benefit the animal by increasing available nutrients for gastrointestinal bacterial populations, which in turn aid in the quantity of nitrogenous waste materials from entering the bloodstream and causing azotaemia. This process is sometimes referred to as nitrogen trapping in renal diets. Examples of prebiotics include:

- **Manno-oligosaccharides (MOS):** This is a prebiotic that also helps to increase the populations of certain microflora that benefit the animal. Its unique structure also attracts pathogens and bonds them to the manno-sugars, rather than attaching to the surface of the gut villi.
- **Glutamine:** This is an amino acid commonly included in critical care nutrition diets, due to its immune-enhancing properties, and ability to enhance wound

healing. Glutamine is utilised in rapidly dividing cells, such as epithelial ente-rocytes and mucosal immune cells. It acts as a prebiotic by maintaining the overall health of the gut lining, and therefore ensuring optimal nutrient absorption.

- **Fructo-oligosaccharides (FOS):** This acts as a nutrient source for the beneficial bacteria of the gastrointestinal tract. It also increases gut transit time, and draws water into the faeces, increasing bulk and softness.

References

Hayek MG, Massimino SP, Michael MS, Ceddia MA. Modulation of immune response through nutraceutical interventions: implications for canine and feline health. *Vet Clin North Am Small Anim Pract* 2004; 34:229–247.

Thorne J. To supplement or not to supplement? Part 1. *VN Times* 2005; Dec:10–11.

14 Rabbit Nutrition

The diet of many rabbits is a direct link to causal effect of ill health, whether it is through poor dentistry or obesity. Life stage diets are now commonly available on the commercial market. All of these diets are designed to be complementary, and fed alongside grass and hay.

Rabbits have a low requirement for fat levels in their diet; 1–2% is ideal. Any fat in the diet should be of vegetable origin; animal fats contain cholesterol that can cause the rabbit to develop atherosclerosis-like symptoms (TeSelle et al. 2012).

A recommended protein level for an adult maintenance diet is 12–14%. Animals that require high energy levels due to physical, environmental and psychological stressors may require a protein level of 16–22%. A fat level of 1% and fibre content of 20% is often quoted.

Changes in the way in which rabbits are now kept should be borne in mind. House rabbits are now commonplace, as is neutering. Neutering has a similar effect on rabbit metabolism as it does in cats and dogs. Rabbit caretakers (this is the preferred terminology, rather than 'owner') should be made aware of this, as obesity can occur, and prevention is better than cure.

There are many different opinions on which vegetables are suitable for rabbits. Most sources agree that carrots, carrot tops, broccoli and parsley are safe, although carrots should only be fed in small amounts because of their high sugar content. Other vegetables that have been used include dandelions, turnip greens, spinach, kale and romaine lettuce. Beans, potatoes and some lettuces are potentially problematic. Recommended guidelines for the amount of vegetables given daily are to feed at least three types of greens daily (along with carrot, if the caretaker wishes to use it). It is important to fed more than one type of vegetable in order to prevent nutrient imbalances. The use of a complementary pelleted diet can aid in reducing any imbalances. Some vegetables (kale, mustard greens and spinach) contain high levels of oxalates. Instead of removing them from the diet altogether, as they are beneficial, their use should be limited to 1–3 meals per week. If you are advising a rabbit caretaker on increasing the vegetable content of the rabbit's diet, it is exceptionally important to advise them to make any changes slowly and also to remind them that vegetables should be washed thoroughly before being offered to

The Consulting Veterinary Nurse, First Edition. Nicola Ackerman.
© 2012 John Wiley & Sons, Ltd. Published 2012 by John Wiley & Sons, Ltd.

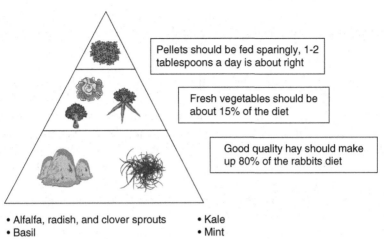

Pellets should be fed sparingly, 1-2 tablespoons a day is about right

Fresh vegetables should be about 15% of the diet

Good quality hay should make up 80% of the rabbits diet

- Alfalfa, radish, and clover sprouts
- Basil
- Beet greens (tops)
- Bok choy
- Broccoli (mostly leaves/stems)
- Brussels sprouts
- Carrot tops
- Celery
- Cilantro
- Clover
- Collard greens
- Dandelion greens (NO pesticides)
- Endive
- Escarole
- Green peppers
- Kale
- Mint
- Mustard greens
- Parsley
- Pea pods (the flat edible kind)
- Peppermint leaves
- Radicchio
- Radish tops
- Raspberry leaves
- Romaine lettuce (NO iceberg or light coloured leaf lettuce)
- Spinach
- Watercress
- Wheat grass

Figure 14.1   Food pyramid showing proportions of foods that should make up a rabbit's diet.

the rabbit. The proportions of diet constituents for the rabbit are usually shown in the form of a feeding pyramid, and this make a good visual aid for rabbit caretakers. (Figure 14.1).

Rabbits should not be fed high-sugar treats such as chocolate drops. Treats for rabbits do exist; examples include small amounts of dried foods such as raisins. These must be fed in very small quantities, but in reality the rabbit does not need them in its diet. Chocolate is poisonous to rabbits and should not be fed, and yoghurt drops have very high sugar content. Other foods that should be avoided include pasta, bread, biscuits, crackers and breakfast cereals.

Young rabbits

Alfalfa can be fed to young bunnies under the age of 6 months since it provides extra calcium necessary for growing bones. It is important to offer timothy hay as well, so when it comes time to wean them to strictly grass hay they will know the taste and be less likely to resist change. Pelleted life stage diets tend to contain higher levels of alfalfa, and thus an increase in calcium levels. Up to the stage of sexual maturity, which tends to be around 6 months of age, a diet containing 16–18% protein, 3% fat and 16–18% fibre is required in order to allow for growth and development.

Young rabbits are only fed once daily by their mother, as the mother's milk is exceptionally high in fat. In the wild, feeding in this manner also reduces the risk of predators locating the nest. The young rabbits will start to be interested in solids at roughly 2 weeks of age, and will consume what the doe is eating. The act of caecotrophy usually starts at around 3 weeks of age. A healthy mixture of greens, hay and pellets is recommended as it will encourage the young rabbits to have a varied diet. Complete weaning occurs at 5–6 weeks of age. When the young are rehomed, it is recommended that they are fed exactly the same diet as when they were with the doe. Any dietary changes must occur very slowly, and the stress of separation can also act as a factor in digestive upset. Any required dietary changes can be made once the young rabbit has completely settled in.

Senior rabbits

The diet of senior rabbits should reflect any clinical problems usually associated with older age. Weight loss commonly occurs, but the causative problem is rarely defined. In some cases the use of alfalfa can be useful as it has a higher energy density and is slightly more enticing to eat than grass hay. Animals with dental problems benefit from vegetables cut slightly smaller, or moistened pellets, in order to aid in an adequate nutrient intake. In cases where the animal appears to be in pain, the use of analgesia should be highly recommended. In many cases it is often ignored by the owner as a consequence of old age.

Dental disease

The diet of rabbits has been blamed for the majority of gastrointestinal and dental disorders. Problems such as myiasis (fly strike) can be attributed to the diarrhoea that the rabbit might have been suffering from. Rabbits' teeth are thought to grow at approximately 3 mm per week. Adequate levels of mastication are required in order to prevent overgrowth of the incisors and molars. Even a slight overgrowth of the rabbit's incisors can cause the alignment of the jaw to alter slightly and this can result in overgrowth of the molars, with spur formation. This problem requires correction via dentistry, but the cause of the tooth overgrowth also needs to be addressed. Client education on the correct types of foods for rabbits is important. The use of coarse mixtures should be avoided, as the animals may select the highly palatable high-sugar pieces, and consequently avoid the healthier high-fibre pieces. If concentrates are to be fed, pellets are recommended, and should only make up a very small portion of the diet. Most of the diet should be made up of hay, grasses and vegetables.

Clinical signs of dental disease in rabbits include:

- Maloccusion causing overgrowth of the teeth, most notably the incisors
- Salivation, commonly noted as a wet chin or dewlap
- Poor body condition
- Appears hungry, but won't eat, or is unable to
- Asymmetrical or lumpy mandibles

Owners should be encouraged to examine their rabbit's teeth on a weekly basis in order to identify any problems.

Creating a soft chewing environment for rabbits can be exceptionally beneficial. Providing objects such as cardboard, wood, dried pinecones, unlaquered wicker baskets and straw mats will aid in maintaining dental health.

Obesity

Obesity in rabbits is starting to become more common. This is mainly due to the inappropriate diets that rabbits are often fed, and to lack of exercise. Obesity and poor diet can be a major causative factor for the development of myiasis. In many cases the rabbit is too large to practice caecotrophy, and the sticky caecotrophs attract flies. Careful dietary modification is needed in these cases. Any dramatic changes in diet, even on to a more nutritious one, will have damaging effects. Dietary changes must occur very slowly. Starvation is not an option in rabbits, due to the chance of inducing hepatic lipidosis. An ideal diet must be low-calorie and high-fibre.

In many cases the removal of all inappropriate foodstuffs and an increase in roughage (grass and hay) and vegetables is all that is required. Low-calorie pelleted diets are available on the market, but these are no substitute for a good all-round balanced diet, combined with exercise.

Chronic renal failure

Symptomatic treatment of clinical signs is the only treatment available for chronic renal failure (CRF), as in other species. As in equines dietary calcium restriction is beneficial, because of the impaired renal excretion of calcium (Harcourt-Brown 2002). Foods such as fresh grass, carrots, apples and cabbage have a moderate to low calcium content, and make them suitable for rabbits suffering from CRF. Foodstuffs such as alfalfa, kale and broccoli have high calcium contents.

Urolithasis

Rabbits excrete higher levels of calcium in their urine than other mammals (Harkness 1994), and this contributes to the cloudiness of the urine. Haematuria can also be incorrectly diagnosed in rabbits. Many rabbit caretakers and uninformed veterinary personnel mistake the presence of orange-to-red coloured by-products in the urine (porphyrinuria) for blood. These by-products result from the normal breakdown of chlorophyll and other vegetable dietary components.

Calcium carbonate crystals are considered normal in the urine, but can easily become a problem when stones are formed. Clinical symptoms of bladder disease and/or bladder stones will vary in each individual, but can include:

- Urine scalding
- Wetness around the genital area
- Semi-solid urine, can be described as toothpaste-like
- Dysuria, demonstrated by hopping in and out of the litter tray/pan, straining and loss of litter training.

Diagnosis can be easily made with radiography and urinalysis, though it should be remembered that rabbits will have some radio-opaque material present in the urine anyway, due to its high calcium content. The only treatment for calcium-containing uroliths is surgery, as the stones cannot be dissolved.

Clinical nutrition

Clinical nutrition for these animals is based on the reduction of calcium in the diet, and perioperative nutrition. This again is dependent on the nutritional status of the individual animal. Lowering blood calcium levels is a simpler process in rabbits than in other mammals. A medium-sized rabbit has a daily minimum requirement of 510 mg of calcium. Alfalfa hay is extremely high in calcium and should not be fed to these animals. The use of grass hays, such as timothy or oat hay, is advocated. Root vegetables are low in calcium, but the majority of vegetables fed to rabbits tend to have high calcium contents. These greens should be limited, but not removed, as they are still a very important component of the diet. Broccoli flowers and stem, dark leaf lettuce, watercress, Brussels sprouts, celery leaves, and cabbage are good choices when trying to reduce calcium. Pelleted diets should also be removed or restricted; pellets designed for young rabbits, or containing alfalfa, should be removed.

References

Harcourt-Brown F. Anorexia in rabbits 2: Diagnosis and treatment. *In practice*. 2002; Sept:450–467.
Harkness JE. Summary of calcium in rabbits. *Rabbit Health News* 1994; 11:7.
TeSelle E, McBee C, Bedown SA. *Natural Nutrition Part II: Pellets and Veggies*. 2012. http://www.rabbit.org/journal/3-4/pellets.html

Part III

Behavioural Issues

15 Puppy and Kitten Behaviour

Puppy and kitten clinics

Clinics for puppies and kittens should start as early as possible. Prevaccination checks are an ideal opportunity to start bonding the client to the practice. Veterinary nurses who are SQPs (see Chapter 1) can prescribe appropriate parasite control for these animals, and provide the owner with useful information. Checklists can be used in order to write recommendations for the owner, and to ensure that all subjects are covered. Vaccination protocols should also be confirmed, as owners sometimes find them confusing.

Ideally these clinics should run monthly from the second vaccination until 6 months of age. The basic purpose is to weigh the animal in order to calculate a correct dose of wormer for the owner to use, though the clinic is an ideal time to offer expert advice on a range of subjects. Topics include nutrition, microchipping, neutering, behaviour, training, socialisation, pet insurance, parasite control and anything else that the owner wishes to discuss. Checklists can be used to ensure that all subjects are covered, and are especially useful when more than one nurse is conducting the clinics: in this way all subjects are covered and any important points are noted.

Socialisation of puppies

Owners who are considering purchasing a new puppy should be encouraged not to take ownership of their puppy until it is at least 8 weeks of age. Earlier than this, and they can lose out on one or several weeks of maternal education and social learning. These puppies might have a higher risk of suffering from emotional disorders later in life.

The role of the veterinary nurse is paramount in educating clients about the importance of puppy socialisation. Veterinary practices should openly promote puppy clinics, puppy parties and socialisation groups. Nurses need to understand the how puppies assimilate these learning processes in order to fully convey to owners why their puppies display certain behaviours.

The Consulting Veterinary Nurse, First Edition. Nicola Ackerman.
© 2012 John Wiley & Sons, Ltd. Published 2012 by John Wiley & Sons, Ltd.

The socialisation period begins at 3 weeks of age and is a period of rapid brain development that coincides with the maturation and myelination of the spinal cord (Shepherd 2002). At this age the puppy becomes fully aware of its environment, and able to respond to it. There are many aspects of socialisation that occur in the main socialisation period (4–14 weeks), but the features of the most long-term behavioural significance are:

- Development of anticipatory responses as a result on an increased ability to attend to the environment
- Emergence of social behaviour
- Ability to form primary social relationships with conspecifics and with other animals (including people).

In puppies up to the age of 5 weeks there is a rapid increase in the tendency to approach unfamiliar people. After 5 weeks puppies become increasingly cautious of unfamiliar individuals or situations, but social motivation to approach and interact outweighs fear up to the age of 8 weeks. From the age of 12–14 weeks puppies are easily frightened, and after 12–14 weeks the growing tendency to react fearfully to novelty puts an end to effective socialisation.

In the juvenile period (14 weeks to sexual maturity) gradual improvement of the motor skills occurs and refinement of behaviour patterns in both relevance and context are seen. During this period there is an increased tendency to explore the environment. At about 4 months of age the speed of formation of conditioned reflexes begins to slow down, as associations made previously probably interfere with new learning. There is evidence for a second period of heightened sensitivity to fear-provoking stimuli just before puberty at around 4–6 months, and an increase in social aggression (Dehasse 1994).

The nurse's role in aiding clients with socialisation of puppies must start from a very early age. Better results can be achieved if socialisation can be started while the puppies are still with the bitch. This is only possible if breeders are open to the idea and take on responsibility for the socialisation of the puppies.

Feeding behaviour when a puppy is with its with littermates can greatly influence its feeding behaviour in adulthood. When with littermates, puppies should have their own food bowl: puppies that have to share a bowl are more likely to bolt their food down (which can result in vomiting if food is eaten too quickly), and more prone to food guarding and thus the potential for obesity in later life.

When puppies are presented to the veterinary practice they are already roughly 8 weeks of age, a period where socialisation is exceptionally important. Nurse clinics are an ideal opportunity to educate owners on why socialisation is required and how to achieve it. Monthly nurse clinics that are tied in with worming regimes present an ideal opportunity to monitor how clients are doing with socialisation, but this may be too late in many cases (Figure 15.1).

A vital role of the veterinary surgeon during the primary vaccination course is to highlight the importance of socialisation to clients, and encourage them to attend puppy socialisation parties. These parties are mainly run by veterinary

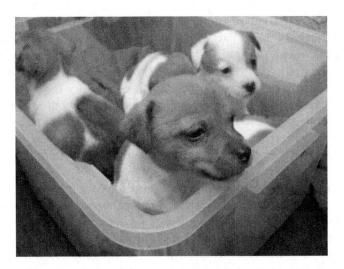

Figure 15.1   Litter of puppies presented to puppy clinic.

nurses and are vital in educating owners on how they are to go about socialising their puppy. It is also important to remember that this is usually the puppy's first visit to the practice, and therefore needs to be as atraumatic as possible and positively pleasant for the puppy. Many books have socialisation charts that can be followed by owners and give a good indication of what they should be attempting to achieve with their puppy. It is important to instil in owners the idea that puppies should be socialised in a wide variety of different ways. People's circumstances can change, and therefore puppies should be socialised in everything that they may possibly encounter in their lives. People who live in rural areas should take their puppies into the city for socialisation, and vice versa. Owners who do not have children still need to socialise their puppy with children, as a new baby may come into the house later on in the dog's life. It is impossible to predict the future and this should be strongly emphasised to owners.

Puppy parties

Puppy parties are now, fortunately, a service almost expected by new puppy owners, and can be a deciding factor for these owners in choosing a specific veterinary practice. Parties need to be orderly and well run, in order not to cause more problems than they prevent.

Deciding on a format for puppy parties

Puppy parties can be an ideal opportunity to bond clients to the practice, but, more importantly, they enable new puppy owners to achieve a well-rounded puppy that can be fully integrated into the family and environmental setting.

Puppy parties can be one-off sessions for the opportunity for puppies to socialise, or a series of parties. One-off parties can be useful and informative for people with limited time to commit to a series of parties, giving a good grounding for owners in how to successfully socialise and habituate their puppies. A series of parties can be in a 'roll on, roll off' format, so that it is not necessary for an owner to wait a new course to start before being able to attend, and therefore missing out on valuable socialising time. A series of parties is ideal for puppies that are a little hesitant to start with when mixing with the other puppies for the first time. This approach gives you a better opportunity to bond clients, as more contact time is achievable.

Before deciding on the format you want to use for your puppy party it is important that you first do a lot of background reading, and gain all of the knowledge that is necessary to run a successful, good-quality puppy party. If you decide on a course of puppy parties, a different topic can be covered each week. Subjects that clients like to have covered include first aid, training issues (including house-training, recalls, play-biting), socialisation and behaviour. As these topics are covered in depth it is important that you give good, knowledgeable and correct information to clients. With new puppies starting each week, you will get many of the same questions having to be answered each week, but this provides an opportunity to reinforce habituation techniques.

Marketing

When the decision has been made to start running puppy parties, everyone in the practice needs to be on board with promoting the benefits. On initial vaccination of the puppy the veterinary surgeon needs to discuss the importance of socialisation, and also to mention the part that puppy parties play in establishing the groundwork for socialising the puppy with other puppies, and with the veterinary practice and its staff.

The puppy parties should be advertised on the practice's website, in any newsletters, in puppy packs that are given out to clients, in waiting room displays – anywhere that be seen by the puppy's owner. Prospective clients ring around veterinary practices to check prices for puppy vaccinations, and promoting the parties at this initial phone call can make a difference to whether that client chooses your practice or not.

Certain parameters need to be set up before you start to promote your parties, and all staff members need to be aware of these so that the correct information is given out. You need to establish an upper age limit on the puppies that can attend the party, and whether they need to have completed their vaccination course or just the first vaccination. Most practices tend to allow only puppies that have had their second vaccination. If you want to include puppies that have not received their full vaccination course, you could always hold a separate one-off puppy party for those that have received just the first part of their vaccination course. If you decide to run a course of parties and the puppy will reach the upper age limit before completing the course, then this is fine. The puppy will still benefit from attending some of the classes, and some are better than none. It is wise to have a maximum number of puppies that can attend the party; if you find that you are oversubscribed then consider providing another course at a different time.

Running the puppy party

A safe, controlled environment is essential when conducting a puppy party. If you decide to use the practice waiting room, it is important that the floor has been cleaned with a viricidal disinfectant, because of the puppies' immature immunological status.

A natural format is to provide seating in a circle (Figure 15.2), but don't be afraid to move people around depending on the nature of their puppy. Having a very boisterous puppy next to a timid puppy is a situation that needs to be avoided.

All information that is given out during the puppy party needs to be accurate, clear and concise. Attending seminars, reading around the subject areas and distance learning is essential, and talking to other nurses who have experience running puppy parties is a valuable resource.

Owners should keep puppies on their leads unless told otherwise, and only a couple should have off-lead time at any one time. The party should never become

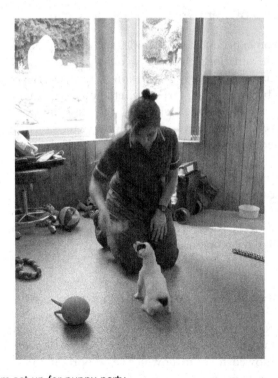

Figure 15.2   Room set up for puppy party.

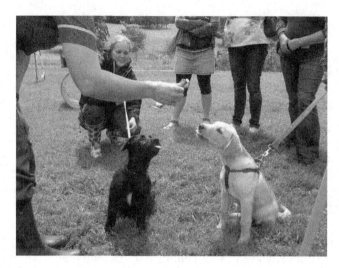

Figure 15.3   Puppies should be kept on leads until specified.

a complete free-for-all. Off-lead time should be structured, with puppies being matched with others of a similar character (Figure 15.3).

Advice to give to owners when things go wrong

Not all socialisation experiences will be positive ones, as one no can foresee a bad situation. Most bad situations cannot be avoided, but clients who are forewarned are forearmed. Running through a situation where the puppy is spooked by a strange object (a bus, a flapping tarpaulin, etc.) and how the owner should react is ideal. Owners should be made aware that the puppy's lead is a means of communication between the handler and the puppy. A nice relaxed lead will help to make the puppy feel relaxed; a tense lead could result in the puppy becoming tense.

Owners should be aware of what to do if the puppy becomes scared. All positive behaviour needs to be rewarded; all negative behaviour should be ignored. If the puppy becomes scared of a bus driving past too closely, this initial reaction should be ignored. When the puppy then starts to act 'normal' again, walking relaxed on the lead, this needs to be rewarded with attention, a toy or treat. Lots of positive experiences will outweigh one negative experience.

What to do if things go wrong during a puppy party

If things do start to get out of hand between two or more puppies during a puppy party, it is important to intervene quickly. The puppies should be put back on to their leads and allowed to calm down. The important thing is to ensure that potentially negative experiences do not occur, and constant monitoring of the

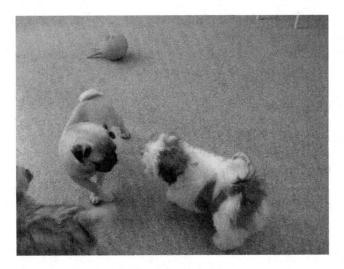

Figure 15.4 It is important not to overwhelm puppies during parties.

puppies' interaction is required. This is a prime reason for not having too many puppies in the party unless you have extra help to monitor them. It can be difficult to monitor the puppies while also answering the owner's questions, and having an additional pair of eyes can be really helpful.

Quiet puppies

There will always be some puppies that are very quiet, cautious or hesitant about interacting with the others when attending puppy parties (Figure 15.4). If there is more than one puppy in the group that is like this, it is best to sit them next to each other away from the more boisterous ones. If there are no suitable puppies to interact with, it can be beneficial for the puppy just to observe for the first session. In order for the puppy not to become too dependent on the owner, the puppy can just observe from your own lap. In most cases, by the end of the session the puppy might be starting to come out a little and might be able to walk around the other puppies (with the others being on their leads).

Training and behaviour

Most training revolves around establishing consequences for the dog's behaviour. Operant conditioning uses these following four types of consequences:

- **Positive reinforcement** adds something to the situation to increase the chance of the behaviour being exhibited again.
- **Negative reinforcement** removes something from the situation to increase the chance of the behaviour being exhibited again.

- **Positive punishment** adds something to the situation to decrease the chance of the behaviour being exhibited again.
- **Negative punishment** removes something from the situation to decrease the chance of the behaviour being exhibited again.

Most trainers claim that they use 'positive training methods'. Generally, this means using reward-based training to increase good behaviour rather than physical punishment to decrease bad behaviour. Operant conditioning deals with the modification of voluntary behaviour or operant behaviour, using the above positive and negative reinforcements and punishments. Punishment here does not mean a physical or verbal punishment, but the removal of something from the environment or situation. For example, when pulling on the lead, the behaviour will result in negative reinforcement, the owner removing speed from the walk – slowing the walk down.

Play-biting

Owners are often worried about play-biting, but the problem can easily be overcome with good instructions. New puppy owners can easily relate to what their puppy was like when it was still amongst its littermates. When one of them played a little too rough with another, the 'hurt' puppy would inform the 'naughty' littermate of this by a loud, high-pitched squeak. The 'hurt' puppy's behaviour straight after the incident would be to completely ignore the 'naughty' puppy, even when the 'naughty' puppy keeps trying to get its attention. When the new owners take their puppy home they need to take over in teaching the puppy social etiquette. If the puppy is starting to play-bite or mouth, the owner needs to imitate the noise that a hurt puppy would make. The most important part is then to ignore the puppy. This includes all forms of communication; the owner should not talk to, look at, or touch the puppy. This can be difficult, especially for younger children, and in some cases the puppy can single out one or two members of the family to target. In these situations, getting the children to stand still with their hands on their heads can help. When explaining this technique to owners it is important to really emphasise the importance of ignoring the puppy after making the high-pitched squeak. With highly boisterous puppies, 'time away' can be used. Separating the puppy from the rest of the family can help; the worst thing in a puppy's world is to be ignored. Distraction techniques can also be used to deflect play-biting behaviour towards play toys rather than towards people.

House-training

Puppy crates are widely used, and can aid in house-training. Advice offered on house-training needs to be consistent from all members of staff. Many pet shops sell 'puppy pads', which are similar to incontinence sheets. These are now being used in place of pieces of newspaper on the floor. This method of house-training can prove to be confusing to puppies, as they are initially trained to urinate on the paper and then are trained not to urinate on the paper but to urinate outside.

Obviously the best time to discuss house-training techniques with owners is as soon as possible, before any inappropriate behaviour becomes learned behaviour. Owners should be encouraged to use a 'key word' when house-training puppies. Most people already use one, but are unaware that they are doing so. Words such as 'toilet' or 'pee-pee' are most commonly used, and need to be used by everyone who comes into contact with the puppy during the house-training process. Puppies need to be taken outside at appropriate times – as soon as the puppy wakes up, after feeding and once the puppy has finished playing. The owner needs to be really aware of what the puppy is doing in order to intervene if required.

Puppies that 'perform' in the appropriate place need to be rewarded. A reward doesn't need to be in the form of food. Rewards are something that an individual perceives as a bonus to their everyday life (Table 15.1); owners need to find which area their pet values the most and use that as a reward. For a terrier a squeaky toy will be ultimately more rewarding than food. When using toys, a toy box is important (Figure 15.5). When all of the dog's toys are lying around the house it

Table 15.1 The four areas of reward

Reward	Examples
Possessions	Toys, favourite types (squeaky, chewy)
Environment	Bed, puppy crate, favourite place to sit
Food	Main diet, treats
Social interactions	Fuss from owners, playing with people and other dogs, grooming

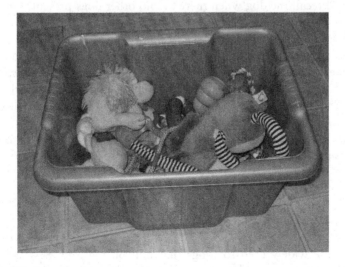

Figure 15.5 Toy boxes.

is less likely to want to play with them. The toys should be placed in a toy box, and one toy brought out at a time and used. Once the dog has finished playing with it, the toy should be put away. Each time the dog has shown any desired behaviour a new toy should be presented to the dog to play with. Depending on the kind of toy this does also include the owner playing with the dog and toy.

Recalling a dog

An ability to recall the dog is one of the most important training skills to be learned. The owner must be able to recall the dog as and when required in order to prevent accidents, and to avoid certain situations. As with all training, it is important to pick a key word that will be used by all the family members, and to use a reward that the dog will rate highly. Start small, by recalling the dog from one side of the room to another, introducing the reward so that the dog learns to associate the recall with a reward. Once the dog is repeating the desired behaviour, start by recalling the dog from different rooms in the house, always rewarding even if the dog does not always respond immediately. The exercise can then be moved to the garden or another safe enclosed area. The use of long lines is ideal for this situation, as they give the owner the security of the dog still being securely attached to a lead (the long line), but the dog feels 'free' as the line is dragging along the floor. Extendable leads do not allow this as there is always a tension in the line between the owner and the dog, unless the extendable lead is locked out at its full length. This purpose of this exercise is to introduce to the dog the key word for the recall, and the process of recall and reward. Performing the recall in the park or similar environment is a very different situation. There are more distractions and smells for the dog to contend with. The owner should expect the dog to come back every time, but setting up the dog to succeed is important. The owner should recall the dog when there are no other dogs present. Only recalling the dog when it is playing with another dog, or in a similar situation, will only lead to the recall being ignored.

The recall exercise should ideally be practised throughout the length of the dog's period of exercise. Leaving it to the end will teach the dog that the recall is associated with going back on to the lead and going home – the ending of the walk, not a desirable thing for the dog. Owners should be encouraged to attach and detach the lead throughout the length of the walk in order to prevent this association. For the recall to work, the dog has to know that the benefit of obeying the command is greater than that of not obeying – chasing another dog or a squirrel, for example.

Pulling on the lead

Headcollars are widely used for dogs that pull on the lead. Several brands are available; the most commonly used are Haltis and Gentle Leaders. A headcollar enables the owner to have a greater degree of control over the dog, and is used to teach the dog to walk calmly on the lead. Then, with conditioning, the dog can ultimately walk calmly on the lead with a normal collar.

- Leave the house calmly. This may need the dog to become desensitised to the lead, headcollar and any other walking equipment such as the owner's walking shoes, coat, etc.
- If the dog becomes excited at any stage, for example when putting on the lead, move back a step, drop the lead and wait until the dog has become calm. Reward the dog when calm, but try not to excite the dog.
- When out of the house, if the dog pulls, gently apply pressure to the collar and/ or headcollar, and slow down your walking speed. The dog will learn that pulling on the lead will actually slow down the process rather than increasing it.
- Continue the walk as soon as the lead becomes slack.
- Continue on the walk as before, praising the dog enthusiastically whenever it achieves the desired walking position and pace.
- Continue with the training until the dog is walking calmly on a consistently slack lead on walks. This may take several days or even weeks depending on the dog.
- Once the dog is happy with walking with the head collar, it can be 'weaned' off it.
  - Start by attaching the lead to the collar rather than the headcollar, with the dog still wearing the headcollar.
  - Reward good behaviour; if the dog starts pulling, then reattach the lead to the headcollar.
  - Slowly extend the length of time where the headcollar is not required. The dog will learn that pulling is an unsuccessful behaviour and learn to walk calmly beside the owner.

Clicker training

Clicker training is a method based on behavioural psychology that relies on marking desirable behaviour and rewarding it.

Any behaviour can be trained with any animal following these three simple steps:

- Achieve the desired behaviour
- Mark the behaviour
- Reinforce the behaviour.

Achieving the desired behaviour can be achieved by shaping, or by setting up the behaviour to be succeeded. Shaping means positioning a reward so that the dog follows the reward into the positioned required. For example, a treat placed above the dog's head, and moved slightly backwards once the dog's nose is up, will move the dog into the sit position as it tries to get the reward. From this position for the dog to lie down, the treat is brought down to the floor. Once the dog successfully repeats 'lie down', 'roll over' can be achieved by placing the reward next to the dog's ear; as the dog moves its head around to get the reward, move the treat slightly over the back of the dog and the dog will roll over to gain the reward.

As in other situations, setting up to succeed is always recommended, and can be used as part of clicker training. Once the dog has learned the behaviour, and can repeat the behaviour, you add in the 'cue'. This can be a word or a visual command, and the same cue should be used by everyone evolved in training the dog. The word doesn't have to express what you want the dog to do. A good example of this is that for dogs that get overexcited when meeting and greeting people, you can use the cue word 'hello' for the command 'sit'. This way, when someone greets the dog, it automatically sits down rather than jumping up. In situations when the dog gets overexcited when people come to the door, the dog should be ignored until calm. Once it is calm then the dog should be rewarded with meeting the person. Once the dog has learned a command, more than one cue word can be used. The dog can understand that either 'sit' or 'hello' requires the same behaviour, to sit down. Both are rewarded in a different manner, one by attention and the other by a treat.

If the dog does not perform the desired behaviour, clicker trainers should not assume that this is 'disobedience'. Instead, they should ask themselves the following questions:

- Does the animal know the meaning of the cue?
- Does the animal know the meaning of the cue in the environment in which it was first taught, but not in the environment in which it was given this time?
- Does the animal sufficiently desire the reward for doing the behaviour?

If any of these questions identify that the dog is not disobeying, the dog owner needs to go back a step in the training, to see where the confusion in the training has arisen from.

Training groups

Many practices find that their clients seek advice on dog trainers for their puppies, as a follow on from puppy socialisation parties. In most cases this means referring clients onto a dog trainer. It can be very difficult to find a dog trainer who gives advice that the practice is happy with. Difficulties can arise when a dog trainer that you have recommended gives advice conflicting with that given by the practice. Some practices offer training classes run by a veterinary nurse, introducing basic training methods. This has the advantages of increasing client loyalty to the practice, generating an income for the practice, and ensuring that the puppies and owners receive good advice.

Frequently asked questions

Why does my puppy eat its own faeces?

Puppies commonly practice coprophagia, and it can be due to attractive food residues in the faeces. The habit can also be acquired when a puppy is being house-trained. If the puppy is badly disciplined when it defecates in the house, it may start consuming the faeces in order to avoid being disciplined. Common practices in order to stop this behaviour include feeding the puppy pineapple, as it makes the faeces very distasteful, and sprinkling chilli powder on the faeces. In some cases where there is a lot of undigested material in the faeces, it is important to advise faecal analysis in order to establish if there are any gastrointestinal abnormalities.

Will castrating my dog calm him down?

The answer is simply no. Castrating a dog will not calm him down. Only good training will. It is also recommended that dogs with confidence issues are also not neutered. The reason for this is that neutering will remove the hormones that supply the only bit of confidence the dog has, and just compound the problem. Some dogs that are classed as aggressive are showing nervous aggression, and therefore behavioural referral should be sought. Temporary chemical castration can be of benefit to see if surgical castration will cause any behavioural changes, while not having a permanent outcome.

Should I get a kitten when I already have a cat?

If you already have a cat(s) and are planning to expand your feline household then the introduction of a newcomer requires some very serious thought. One consideration is the age of your current cat as well as the new addition. Social maturity in cats is reached between 2 and 3 years of age, and their social tolerance is therefore greater before that age than it is after it. This means that the introduction process is often easier if the resident is less than 2 years of age and the newcomer is also of a similar or a younger age. If the current cat is elderly it is not only social compatibility that needs to be considered but also differing requirements for playful interaction. Young cats have a far higher desire for social play and an elderly cat may find the playful attention too stressful.

References

Dehasse J. Sensory, emotional and social development of the young dog. *Bull Vet Clin Ethol* 1994; 2(1–2): 6–29.

Shepherd K. Development of behaviour, social behaviour and communication in dogs. In: Horwitz D, Mills D, Heath S, eds., *BSAVA Manual of Canine and Feline Behavioural Medicine*. Gloucester: BSAVA Publications, 2002, pp. 8–20.

16 Noise Phobias and Fireworks

Noise phobias in animals can be extremely distressing for both the animal and the owner. In some surveys up to 49% of dog owners reported that their dog had a fear of loud noises. This is a significant number of animals, and therefore a problem that time and effort needs to be invested in. Prevention is always better than cure, but in many cases owners are unaware of the length of time and amount of commitment they will require to help pets with phobias. The education of pet owners is paramount, and an important role for veterinary nurses in practice.

Owners should be informed of the behaviours that they could possibly experience from their pet. They should be told to ignore any fearful behaviour from their pet. Dogs are very intuitive, and can easily pick up on an owner's anxiety. Cats prefer to cope on their own, and should be left in a secure environment. An animal's emotional and stress responses are a normal adaptive response to any kind of stimulus. This enables the animal to deal with variety and change in the environment. The response to stimuli depends on:

- Genetic factors
- Experiences during development
- The success or otherwise of previous responses to the stressor.

This highlights the requirement for noise/firework desensitisation during puppyhood/kittenhood, and the importance of the owner's response in managing

The Consulting Veterinary Nurse, First Edition. Nicola Ackerman.
© 2012 John Wiley & Sons, Ltd. Published 2012 by John Wiley & Sons, Ltd.

any ongoing problems. The prevention of noise phobias should be introduced as a subject in puppy clinics and socialisation classes. Noise phobia/firework CDs can be used as part of habituation programmes for young puppies, under guidance from a knowledgeable person.

General advice around the firework period

In animals that develop noise phobias, the experience of fireworks can be traumatic. Behaviours can range from attention-seeking up to destructive behaviours and inappropriate toileting. It is important in the run-up to any firework events that a management plan has been put into place. Many medication combinations need to be started at least 2 weeks before the event for the full benefit (see Table 16.1).

The pet needs to become accustomed to the use of a bolt-hole. In many cases, if the animal has had a previous bad experience with fireworks they may have already shown where they prefer to hide – under the TV cabinet or behind the sofa, for example. Making a 'den' for the animal there can be highly beneficial (Figure 16.1). A suitable-sized puppy crate with a blanket over the top is ideal (see box). Spraying the den with pheromone spray or use of a plug-in pheromone should be highly recommended. Plug-ins should be plugged in at least 24 hours before you need them. Placing blankets in the crate that the dog can bury itself under and dig around in is also useful (see Box 16.1).

Box 16.1   Making a bolt-hole

- Choose a place that the dog already has a tendency to use
- The dog must have access to this area at all times
- Using a crate as a bolt-hole is ideal
- Piles of blankets to hide under
- Windows shut, heavy curtains drawn to black out light
- Items of the owner's clothing carrying their body odour placed in the bolt-hole
- Background music playing to block out external noise
- A DAP diffuser installed close to the dog's resting place in the bolt-hole

---

You should recommend to owners that all dogs are exercised before nightfall. Dogs that are likely to bolt if they hear a firework should be kept on a lead at all times during the firework season.

With cats, ensure that the animal remains indoors, and any windows and cat flaps are closed. Cats should be used to using a litter tray, as they can become distressed if not habituated to using one. This may predispose to other stress responses such as FLUTD, especially if the cat is reluctant to urinate. Litter trays may need to be placed in areas that the cat is happiest about.

Table 16.1 Pharmaceuticals commonly used in the treatment of noise phobias and anxieties

Drug	Condition best treated	Dosage (oral)		Comments
		Dogs	Cats	
Alprazolam	Panic, profound noise phobias	0.01–0.1–0.25 mg/kg as needed, not to exceed 4 mg/dog/day unless large dog; start at 0.125 mg for 20 kg dog at least 1 h before expected noise; repeat 15 min before and then as needed	0.125–0.25 mg/cat bid–tid	Drug tolerance and dependence may develop
Diazepam	Milder noise reactions or when slightly more of a sedative effect is desirable	0.5–2.2 mg/kg every 4–6 h as needed	0.2–0.4 mg/kg sid–bid or as required	Rare cases of acute liver failure associated with treatment in cats
Amitriptyline	Mild generalised anxieties	2.2–4.4 mg/kg sid or divided bid	5–10 mg/cat sid–bid	Anticholinergic and sedative side effects
Propranolol	Anxiety and fear	0.5–2 mg/kg tid or as required	0.2–1 mg/kg orally	Bradycardia possible side effect. Can be used in combination with phenobarbital
Fluoxetine	Explosive impulsive acts whether associated with anxiety or aggression	0.5–2.0 mg/kg sid	0.5–1 mg/kg sid	Inappetence and anorexia common side effects, especially in higher doses

Bid; twice a day; sid, once a day; tid, three times a day.

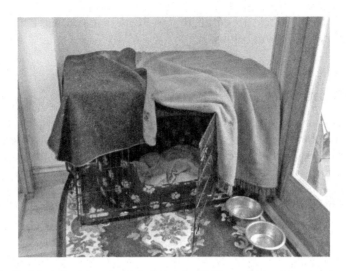

Figure 16.1 Bolt-holes are important in firework phobias.

Microchipping should be recommended for all animals, and can prove especially beneficial if the animal escapes and becomes frightened. Some dogs can find going outside very stressful, even during the day, and the use of pheromone collars can help in reducing anxiety in these animals.

Draw the curtains; turn on the TV or music. But remember to keep to a normal routine; if you only play a specific piece of music during firework season, dogs will pick up on this. It is also important to take into consideration where speakers are placed (not too close to the dog), and that the beat of the music is not too similar to that of the fireworks. These factors are also really important when using desensitisation CDs.

Veterinary practices are well placed to give owners the correct information for helping them and their pets. The difficulty is getting them to ask for this information: many owners are unaware that veterinary practices are able to help in these situations. Many practices mail out information to all clients who have received or requested medication for fireworks, by using searches on the practice's computer system. Searching for words in the clinical text such as 'fireworks', 'phobias', can be done if your practice management system allows. It is less useful to search for the word 'noise', as this word is used when describing respiratory noise, etc.

Client evenings on this topic are always popular and should be timed for the end of the summer; this then gives adequate time for noise desensitisation programmes to be instigated. Client handouts can be prepared, and the local newspaper can also be used in informing owners of the strategies that can be put into place to help animals.

Just remember to stock up on all the products that you want to recommend before the firework season begins.

Phobia treatment

For owners who want to go down the route of behaviour therapy, it must be made clear that this often means altering their own behaviour. This includes ceasing to reward the animal's phobic response; this is usually done inadvertently and is therefore difficult to control. The owner must be willing to participate in a passive behaviour modification programme. Behaviour modification exercises include systematic desensitisation and counter-conditioning, relaxation therapy, encouraging deferential behaviour, crating and siting of safe areas.

Treatment can be summarised as:

- Providing the dog with opportunities to fully develop a reliable coping strategy
- Limiting the effects of further noise exposure
- Use of controlled exposure to the phobic stimulus to reduce future phobic responses
- Use of long-term drug therapy to alter baseline emotional responses to noise events (Bowen 2007).

The basis of therapy is desensitisation and counter-conditioning. In phobia cases the desensitisation is performed in advance of the counter-conditioning. The animal must be aware of the noise, and able to cope with it, before then being able to associate a new, pleasant response to it.

Pheromone use

Pheromones are chemicals released from the surface of the body into the surrounding environment, which affect the behaviour of other individuals (they are normally species specific). There are currently two commercial formulations of pheromone therapy for cats and one for dogs. The two cat pheromones (Feliway and Felifriend, Ceva Animal Health) use different pheromones that help in the reduction of spraying, and lower intercat aggression (Feliway) and in encouraging cats to approach unfamiliar people and aid in handling of cats (Felifriend). Pheromones used for dogs have been identified from the mammary region of the dam shortly after giving birth. These chemicals play a role in the emotional development of young and have been called appeasing pheromones. Dog appeasing pheromone has a calming effect on puppies. It has also been isolated from the ears in some adult dogs, and may play a role in social communication and cohesion. Dog appeasing pheromone (Adaptil, Ceva Animal Health) can play a role in helping reduce aversion to novelty (Figure 16.2).

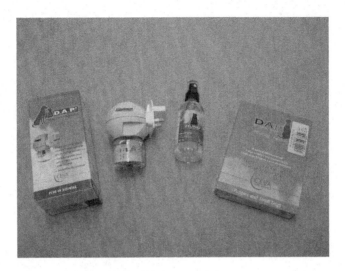

Figure 16.2 Pheromones available in veterinary practice.

Reference

Bowen J. Canine sound phobias. In: *BSAVA Scientific Proceedings Veterinary Programme* 2007, pp. 193–196.

Part IV

'Well Pet' Clinics

17 Vaccination Clinics

Vaccinations are one of the most important forms of preventive medicine in veterinary practice. The vaccine consultation is an opportunity to discuss many matters with a client who may only present the animal to the veterinary practice once a year.

The importance of vaccination

Vaccines work by modifying a viral or bacterial microorganism into a preparation that, when introduced into an animal, stimulates the animal's immunity, but does not produce the same level of clinical symptoms or disease as the original microorganism. Antibodies are produced in the body in response to the antigen (the vaccine) and combine with the antigen to create an antibody–antigen complex. This complex aids in:

- Preventing bacteria attaching to mucosal surfaces
- Neutralising toxins
- Preventing viruses from entering cells
- Activating complement
- Making phagocytosis easier.

The activation of complement factors has a positive effects, as it increase inflammation, thus increasing the number of neutrophils and therefore phagocytosis. Once the antigen has been successfully eliminated, the antibody titre will gradually fall. Some of the B-lymphocytes will then become memory cells specific to the vaccine antigen.

This immune response will only last for a variable period which varies depending on the immunogenicity of the particular vaccine used. Vaccine manufacturers give guidelines for when vaccination boosters are required, in order to maintain a high level of immunity within the animal in case of re-infection.

The Consulting Veterinary Nurse, First Edition. Nicola Ackerman.
© 2012 John Wiley & Sons, Ltd. Published 2012 by John Wiley & Sons, Ltd.

Annual clinical examination

The annual booster consultation of any animal – cat, dog or rabbit – is not just the injection of a vaccine. Before receiving the vaccine, the animal needs a full clinical examination to ensure that it is fit enough to receive the vaccine antigens. This ensures that its immunological status is not compromised by a sudden increase of antigen that it might not be well enough to cope with. Some owners question the requirement for annual vaccinations, and in these cases blood antibody titre levels can be measured in order to see if the vaccination booster is in fact needed. Most veterinary laboratories offer blood screening for this purpose.

It is vital that the annual vaccination is marketed to clients as the annual clinical examination and vaccination. The length of time for this appointment and its set-up is very much dependent on the veterinary practice. Some practices offer a 10 minute appointment, some 20 minutes. In some practices the annual vaccination appointment is split into two parts: an initial consultation with the veterinary surgeon, which includes the clinical examination and administration of the vaccine, followed by an equally long consultation with the veterinary nurse. The nurse's consultation period can be used to give advice on a number of different aspects (endo- and ectoparasite control, dentistry, behaviour, nutrition) and can help to enhance the animal's health status. Other procedures such as nail clipping, blood sampling and blood pressure monitoring can be done at this time too.

Ethics of vaccination

Under Schedule 3 of The Veterinary Surgeons Act 1966, only veterinary surgeons are permitted to administer annual vaccines (boosters) or primary courses. Veterinary nurses are permitted to administer second parts of vaccines, delegated by the veterinary surgeon and working under directions from the veterinary surgeon.

18 Post-Neutering Clinics

After neutering there is a gap of usually up to 8 months until the animal is next seen at its first annual booster (at 14–15 months of age). There is traditionally a fall-off in the number of animals that are seen at their first booster vaccination, and an interim visit between neutering and the vaccination can help prevent this. A clinic aimed at roughly 9 months of age can fill this gap. Attaching a reminder to all neutering procedures for a post-neutering clinic 3 months after surgery will ensure that clients receive a reminder for these clinics. Animals will usually require some form of worming control at roughly 9 months of age, as most are wormed monthly until 6 months of age, and then 3 monthly after this. It is also important to weight the animal and measure its BCS, in order to check that there has not been a large increase in body weight. It is also important to remember that in large breeds of dogs these animals are still growing and therefore monitoring growth rate throughout, until adulthood, is beneficial.

Advice can be given on dietary matters at this clinic. Some animals will have reached maturity by 9 months, and therefore can transition on to adult diets, whereas some need to remain on a puppy diet for longer.

Many diets specifically designed for neutered cats have now been introduced to the market. The animal's metabolism decreases in the period immediately after neutering. In entire cats energy expenditure in both female and male animals is 57 ± 2 kcal/kg. Once neutered, this value decreases to 50 ± 3 kcal/kg in males, and 51 ± 2 kcal/kg in females. Discussion on diet at this stage can reduce the incidence of animals being overweight or obese later in life. There are, however, marked differences in other factors, as demonstrated in Table 18.1. Changes in insulin resistance can suggest predisposition of neutered cats to diabetes mellitus.

The Consulting Veterinary Nurse, First Edition. Nicola Ackerman.
© 2012 John Wiley & Sons, Ltd. Published 2012 by John Wiley & Sons, Ltd.

Table 18.1   Differences between male and female cats, and the consequences of neutering

Parameter	Male	Female	Consequence of neutering
Body fat (as % of total body weight)	23.8 ± 1	30.1 ± 1.7	Increase: M: 32.9 ± 1.7 F: 35.5 ± 1.8
Energy expenditure(kcal/kg)	57 ± 2	57 ± 2	Decrease: M: 50 ± 3 F: 51 ± 2
Non-esterified fatty acids		Higher in the female	Greater differences between males and females
Caloric requirements			Requirements reduced in both sexes
Serum leptin	Regulation of leptin secretion by testosterone	No demonstrated oestrogenic control in cats	M: Increase F: Less noticeable change
Glucose intolerance		Absent	Unchanged in both sexes
Insulin	More marked		M: Continuance of high insulin resistance F: Appearance of insulin resistance

Source: Dethioux et al. (2005).

Reference

Dethioux F, Marniquet P, Petit P, Weber M. How can we prevent the metabolic consequences of neutering? *Focus Special Edition: Preventative nutrition for major health risks in cats* 2005: 9–18.

19 Senior Pet Clinics

Senior pet clinics are notoriously difficult to set up, whether this is due to a general apathy in pet owners when their pet is older, or rather to owners not wanting to take an apparently healthy older pet to the veterinary practice, only for professionals to find something wrong. Senior pet clinics should be marketed more as an aid towards preventive health care and improving quality and longevity of life in older pets. Senior clinics can be either nurse led or vet lead, and either priced to cover all costs or considered as a loss leader. Clinics that are nurse led and offered as a loss leader tend to be more successful.

Senior clinics traditionally cover a full clinical history, clinical examination, blood testing, urine testing and in cats blood pressure monitoring. If these diagnostics are costed out, such clinics can potentially be very expensive. In clinics that are performed as a loss leader, the initial consultation and examination is performed at a discounted rate, or free of charge. The reasoning is that the initial consultation will bring in additional work, e.g. dental procedures, blood testing, urine testing, and blood pressure monitoring. Several studies have noted that the prevalence of dental disease and arthritis (especially in cats) is approximately 80% of all animals over the age of 8 years of age, and therefore the likelihood of 'finding' something is fairly high. Even with completely healthy animals, advice on senior diets, preventive dental care, and making owners aware of which clinical symptoms to be looking out for in their pet is important.

A detailed clinical history needs to be taken from each owner, and this includes behavioural questioning alongside questions relating to feeding patterns, etc. Nurses are in an ideal position to question owners about their pets as in some cases they will speak more freely with nurses than with the veterinary surgeon.

Advising on senior diets

The senior or geriatric phase of life starts at varying ages due to breed size and species. Toy and small breed dogs enter the senior stage of life at approximately

The Consulting Veterinary Nurse, First Edition. Nicola Ackerman.
© 2012 John Wiley & Sons, Ltd. Published 2012 by John Wiley & Sons, Ltd.

8 years, medium breeds at 7–8 years, with large and giant breeds entering a senior life stage at 5 years. Cats are deemed to be senior from 8 years. Other factors such as nutritional status, environment, genetic make-up and clinical health will effect these ages and the longevity of the animal. Changes that occur with age include greying of the muzzle and slowing down in activity levels; less obvious changes include alteration in the physiology of the digestive tract, immune system, kidneys and other organs. Generally, the capacity to absorb and utilise nutrients is not decreased in older animals, but the body does become less able to tolerate excesses and borderline deficiencies and the ability to respond to dietary changes may also be decreased (Morris et al. 2000). 'Geriatric' screening should be considered in all animals once they have reached a senior age. A critical part of this screening should include evaluation of nutrition.

Nutritional changes in cat and dog diets are aimed at supporting the physiological changes that occur within this life stage. Energy requirements for senior animals are reduced, due to a decrease in activity levels and expenditure. Some active senior animals may require an energy density higher than that provided by senior diets, and a compromise between senior and adult maintenance is required.

In cats, however, the maintenance energy requirements do not decrease as the animal gets older (Laflamme 2005), perhaps because cats remaining relatively inactive throughout its adult life. It is difficult to distinguish between an older and a younger cat simply by looking at their activity levels, as cats spend a large portion of their day sleeping. The proportion of obese cats tends to increase until the age of 7, but after this it decreases, especially from the age of 10 years (Dethioux et al. 2005).

A reduction in renal function should be considered in all senior animals. A reduction in the quantity of protein in the diet could be beneficial if renal damage has occurred. The quality of the protein should be increased as skeletal muscle mass reduces, which also reduces any protein or amino acid reserves if required. Some life stage diets do not have decreased protein levels, as some opinions are that restricted protein levels are not required until there is direct evidence of renal impairment. In fact protein requirements sufficient to support protein turnover actually increase in older dogs and cats. Protein restriction in feline senior diets should be avoided. Cats are especially sensitive to decreases in protein levels in the diet because of their inability to downgrade protein metabolism pathways. Reduced protein digestibility is also experienced in geriatric cats. In healthy adult cats protein digestibility is typically 85–90%, but in geriatric cats this digestibility can be reduced to less than 77% (Kelly et al. 2006). Diets with a severely restricted protein level or proteins of a low quality or biological value (BV) can predispose cats over 12 years to negative nitrogen balance, and loss of lean body mass (Kelly et al. 2006).

The restriction of phosphorus in the diet plays a significant role in the prevention of renal impairment. A decrease in kidney function can also lead to an increased loss of the water-soluble vitamins, due to the kidney's decreased ability to concentrate the urine. This can also lead to a reduction in the animal's hydration levels. Senior animals have a reduced sensitivity to thirst, and thus there is a greater risk of dehydration in these animals (Morris et al. 2000).

Most senior diets are formulated to have softer kibbles in order to accommodate any dental problems, reduction in number of teeth, and a decrease in musculature of the jaw. Moving to a moist diet can benefit an animal that is having difficulties in mastication. A moist diet will also aid hydration levels.

The use of antioxidants for senior animals has been advocated, as free radical production can increase with age, as diseases associated with ageing (cardiovascular, arthritis) increase production of free radicals. Older cats and dogs should be evaluated for vitamin and mineral deficiencies. Due to oxidative damage, the demand for antioxidant vitamins (water-soluble vitamins) is greater. Geriatric animals, especially cats, also have a reduced ability to digest fats, and for this reason deficiencies of other essential nutrients (fat-soluble vitamins) can occur (Laflamme 2005).

As the animal ages, smell is the first sense to decline. As the animal's sense of smell deteriorates, it may eat less. Aroma is particularly important in diets aimed at senior animals, in order to encourage consumption.

References

Dethioux F, Marniquet P, Petit P, Weber M. How can we prevent the metabolic consequences of neutering? *Focus Special Edition: Preventative nutrition for major health risks in cats* 2005, pp. 9–18.

Kelly M, Jean-Phillippe C, Cupp C. Advances in nutritional care of the older cat. *VN Times* 2006; June:8–9.

Laflamme DP. Nutrition for ageing cats and dogs, and the importance of body condition. *Vet Clin North Am Small Anim Pract* 2005; 35:713–742.

Morris JG, Rogers QR, Fascetti AJ. Nutrition of healthy dogs and cats in various stages of adult life. In: Hand MS, Thatcher CD, Remillard RL, Roudebush P, eds. *Small Animal Clinical Nutrition*, 4th Edition. Topeka, KS: Mark Morris Institute, 2000, pp. 555–560.

Part V

Medical Clinics

20 Arthritis

Osteoarthritis (OA) can be an exceptionally painful and crippling disease. OA or degenerative joint disease (DJD) is a chronic progressive disease characterised by pathological changes of the movable joints (Figure 20.1). Dietary manipulation can aid in the management of arthritis, and help improve the animal's mobility. Arthritis can be classified into two types:

- Degenerative arthritis, in which the degradation of the articular cartilage is a prominent feature
- Inflammatory arthropathies, where synovitis is the main pathological feature.

OA is the most common form of arthritis experienced in both animals and humans. Management of OA includes weight control, appropriate exercise management and anti-inflammatory medications. OA is characterised by degeneration of the articular cartilage and proliferation of new bone.

Nurse clinics for arthritis

The nurse clinic plays an important part in helping the owner to improve the quality of life for the pet. There are several aspects that owners may need guidance on, along with compliance with any pharmaceuticals that the veterinary surgeon may have prescribed. With the multiplicity of drugs and alternative treatments in use for chronic pain, management of these patients can be difficult and complex. It is important to emphasise to the owners of these pets that multiple trials may be required to find the right combination of analgesics, supplements and diets, and that not all patients can be effectively managed.

The aims of the nursing clinic are to:

- Perform pain scores in order to assess any improvements or deteriorations in arthritic pain
- Aid the client in compliance with pharmaceutical administration
- Advise on a good balanced diet, with correction of any dietary imbalances, including obesity

The Consulting Veterinary Nurse, First Edition. Nicola Ackerman.
© 2012 John Wiley & Sons, Ltd. Published 2012 by John Wiley & Sons, Ltd.

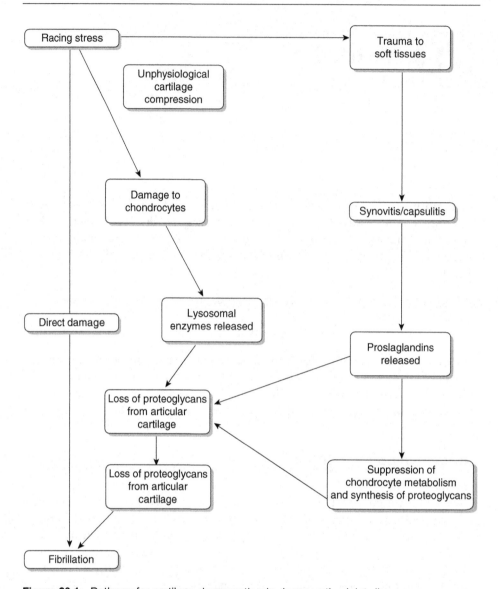

Figure 20.1   Pathway for cartilage degeneration in degenerative joint disease.

- Advise on exercise levels and activities
- Give the client guidance on alternative therapies in order to help the pet's mobility.

Monitoring of arthritic patients

Animals with chronic pain should be rechecked frequently to assess response to therapy and monitor for side effects, and the owners should be consulted closely as to the effectiveness of treatment. All patients that are going to start on a course of analgesics should undertake blood sampling in order to ascertain renal and liver function. Medications such as non-steroidal anti-inflammatory drugs (NSAIDs) can affect hepatic and renal function. Routine blood screening should be done every 6 months while the animal is receiving the medications. Monitoring of urine specific gravity can prove valuable in the early identification of renal insufficiency.

For those animals that have been identified as being arthritic, but have not yet started on any form of treatment, pain scoring should be performed. Although the scoring system is subjective, if the same person performs the scoring before and after treatment it will give a good indication of whether the treatment has worked and to what degree.

Obesity is a major risk factor of OA. Weight loss must be initiated as soon as possible. Exercising and consequently weight loss can be difficult because of restrictions in mobility. A diet for an animal with OA needs to meet the requirements for the animal's life stage and body condition score (BCS).

Arthritis in cats

It has been long assumed that cats, unlike other species, seldom suffer from arthritis, but research has shown that they do. Arthritis is a painful degenerative condition, but the signs exhibited can be very subtle in cats. It has been reported that 90% of cats over the age of 12 years old show changes in their bones suggesting arthritis when they are X-rayed. Being able to recognise whether a cat is suffering from arthritic changes is important, and educating clients on these signs is essential. Slowing down in old age is not an inevitable fact, but rather a possible sign of arthritis, which can be treated. As mentioned, the clinical signs are very subtle, as cats are very good at hiding their pain. In order to ascertain whether the cat is suffering from arthritis, there are lots of very easy signs that the owner can look for. These questions can be presented in a form of a questionnaire that clients can read through before the consultation so that they are already bearing the possibility of arthritis in mind. The questions can include:

- Does your cat appear stiff or lame?
- Have there been any weight changes, either gain (through not getting enough exercise) or loss (loss of appetite due to pain)?
- Have you noticed any change in temperament? Some cats can become very clingy and demand attention, some can become reclusive (this is due to chronic pain), and some can become aggressive.
- Have you noticed any changes in sleep pattern, both increases and decreases? This can be due to not being able to settle (fidgeting) due to pain, or increases due to the exhaustion of pain.
- Has the cat changed where it sleeps? This can indicate pain, as the animal is trying to get comfortable by sleeping on softer areas or may not be able to reach up to its usual sleeping areas.

- Has the cat shown a reduced ability to jump up and down from surfaces, chairs, steps, etc.?
- Have you noticed any changes in toileting behaviour? This can be due to pain and reduced mobility, making climbing into the litter tray undesirable or difficult. Some cats can have difficulty getting through the cat flap in order to reach a toileting area outside.
- Have you noticed a reduction in coat condition, due to reduced grooming activities?
- Have you noticed a frequent licking of joints, due to pain in the joints?
- Has there been a reduction in hunting activities?
- Does the cat have longer claws, due to reduction in scratching (either on a scratching post or on surfaces outside)?

If the owner notices any of these signs in their cat, it should be checked over by the veterinary surgeon.

Diet

Where weight gain has occurred, it is important that the excess weight is lost as this will greatly impact on the cat's mobility. Weight loss can be achieved with a weight loss programme, feeding diets low in calories. There are also diets specifically for cats with arthritis; these can range up to veterinary prescription diets. Where the food is placed should also be considered. Cats that have difficulty jumping will benefit from their food being placed at a lower level. The food still needs to be placed in a place that the cat will feel secure to eat in.

Pain relief

Pain medications are available for cats with arthritis; they are easy to administer (as liquid on the food), and highly effective. Arthritis is a very painful condition, even if your cat does not seem to be in a great deal of pain. Medications will require a veterinary prescription from a veterinary surgeon after a clinical examination.

Acupuncture

Cats, like dogs and rabbits, accept acupuncture treatment well, and it does make a difference to the pain levels that the pet is suffering from. Most owners report that their pet seemed happier after treatments (Figure 20.2).

Touch therapy and grooming

Some grooming mitts can also be used as massage groomers, as can Zoom Grooms. Massage and touch is readily accepted by some cats.

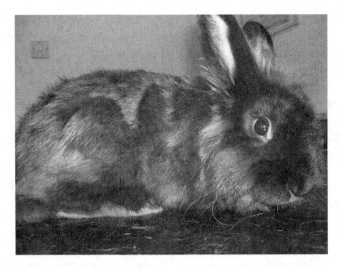

Figure 20.2   Acupuncture in a rabbit.

Environmental enrichment

Cats prefer a place where they can climb up and sit. Cats suffering from arthritis will find this difficult, and this will reduce the number of places for them to sit and hide away, especially from other family members (children and other pets). Owners can provide more hiding places: igloos and cat pouches are popular. Some arthritic cats prefer warmth, and a warm bed is especially appreciated.

If the cat is having problems with toileting, it may be because they feel more vulnerable when in the tray. Moving the litter tray to a more private area or getting a covered tray can help. Cats like to have more than one 'escape' route from their territory (the house). If they are unable to jump from lower windows as they used to do, or if they now find using the cat flap more difficult, thought should be given to alternative routes for them. This can include using ramps to lower windows, or larger and differently designed cat flaps.

Nutraceuticals

Nutraceuticals are nutrients that are administered at a high enough level to have positive effects in the body. The main nutraceuticals used for arthritis are glucosamine hydrochloride and chondroitin sulphate. These can be obtained in many different forms and in different strengths. Some diets already contain these supplements, but care should be given to the way in which the supplements are made and the source of the additives. Price gives an indication of the quality of the supplement. If the animal is insured, supplements obtained from a veterinary practice can sometimes be claimed for.

Oils can also be used to aid with arthritis; cod liver oil has been traditionally used. These oils contain omega fatty acids; they can also be obtained in more concentrated forms than cod liver oil, and in some diets.

The use of chondroprotectants and other nutraceuticals has become commonplace for cats and dogs suffering from OA. Chondroprotective agents are reported to have three primary effects:

- Anabolic: supports or enhances metabolism of chondrocytes and synoviocytes
- Catabolic: inhibits degradative enzymes within the synovial fluid and cartilage matrix
- Antithrombolic: inhibits the formation of thrombi in small blood vessels supplying the joint (Beale 2004).

Nutraceuticals are a type of chondroprotective agents and are defined as non-drug substances that are produced in a purified or extracted form and administered orally to provide compounds required for normal body structure and function, with the intent of improving health and well-being. Different types of nutraceuticals used in the management of OA are described below.

Fatty acids

Eicosapentaenoic acid (EPA) is the most effective omega-3 (n-3) polyunsaturated fatty acid (PUFA) for preventing cartilage catabolism in *in vitro* models. This data suggests that supplementation of food with EPA should prove to be beneficial in slowing the rate of cartilage degradation in canine degenerative joint disease (DJD). EPA blocks the genes that produce cartilage-destroying enzymes, aggrecanase and matrix metalloproteinases (MMPs). These enzymes cause progression of the disease, which continues even in the absence of inflammation; for example, if the animal is medicated with NSAIDs. NSAIDs stop the inflammation that is caused by chondrocyte damage but this does not stop degradation. The symptoms of OA are being controlled but as the damage is continuing gradual increases in medication will be required. EPA is the only omega-3 fatty acid that is taken up by chondrocytes and remains active within the joint. EPA also helps soothe the inflammation associated with OA (Figure 20.3). Use of diets enriched with EPA have shown that the dose of NSAIDs required to control clinical signs in dogs with OA could be reduced (Beale 2004).

The ratio of fatty acids is of great importance. High levels of omega-3 to omega-6 are required. This differs greatly from the ratios of fatty acids previously used for inflammation processes, e.g. atopy. Alpha-linolenic acid (ALA) is often added to canine diets, as it is a precursor to EPA.

Glucosamine

Glucosamine supplements are the most commonly used in the OA market, and glucosamine hydrochloride and glucosamine sulphate are the most commonly

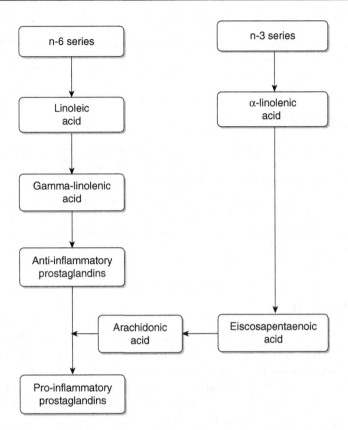

Figure 20.3 Inhibition of inflammatory pathways by supplementation of EPA.

found. Of the two, glucosamine hydrochloride will yield more glucosamine per unit weight to the animal than the sulphate form. This should be clearly explained to the owner, who may wish to purchase non-veterinary products that appear cheaper. Glucosamine is a precursor to glycoaminoglycans (GAGs), which are present in the extracellular matrix of articular cartilage. When damage to chondrocytes occurs there is a decreased ability to synthesise glucosamine. Supplementing the diet stimulates the production of proteoglycans and collagen by these cells.

In traumatic DJD, the natural balance between synthesis and degradation of cartilage shifts towards increasing degradation, resulting in loss of mucopolysaccharides. Commercially used products are chemically similar to the mucopolysaccharides of the articular cartilage, and are concentrated into the cartilaginous tissue. Polysulphated glycoaminoglycan (PSGAG) has been available for many years, and is routinely used as an intra-articular therapy for equine joint disease. PSGAG has a potent ability to inhibit various lysosomal enzymes associated with proteoglycan breakdown. Some PSGAGs have been shown to be a potent inhibitor of degrading enzymes of cartilage, and stimulate the metabolism of chondrocytes and synovial cells. Experimental work with PSGAG has indicated the prevention of further progressive degeneration within the joint in postsurgical cases. This fact is particularly important when considering possible prophylactic schemes, especially for young animals in training.

Chondroitin sulphate

Chondroitin sulphate (CS) is another GAG present within the extracellular matrix of the articular cartilage. CS has been shown to stimulate the production of proteoglycans and collagen like glucosamine, but can also inhibit histamine-mediated inflammation, decrease interleukin-1 production and inhibit metalloproteinases. Experimental use of oral and intramuscularly CS in induced equine arthritis has shown that a decrease in articular cartilage was present, suggesting a direct anti-inflammatory effect of CS on the injury caused (May 1996).

Sodium hyaluronate

The mode of action of sodium hyaluronate (SH) is unknown, but binding to the cartilage proteoglycans may slow the process of cartilage degradation, and the increase in synovial fluid viscosity may also prove to be beneficial. SH exerts an anti-inflammatory action by inhibiting the movement of granulocytes and macrophages. SH has been described as a treatment for DJD, and has shown to be useful with synovitis, but not when obvious cartilage degeneration is present (McIlwraith and Vachon 1998).

Postoperative use of chondroprotectants

All surgery performed on any joint will induce some level of OA. The use of chondroprotectants has been encouraged in the postoperative period and during physical rehabilitation period to accelerate and enhance recovery. Periods of immobilisation should be discouraged, as reduction in synovial fluid production and proteoglycan depletion occurs due to the reduction in loading on the joint. The use of chondroprotectants aids in pain relief, so that the animal is more likely to perform physiotherapy exercises: it reduces the degradative and inflammatory enzymes which help protect the cartilage and stimulates the synovial fluid, proteoglycan and collagen production to promote cartilage matrix repair.

A multimodal approach needs to be taken when considering treatments for OA. Nutritional therapy and analgesia are only two; other therapies such as acupuncture, hydrotherapy, magnetic collars and modified exercise regimes should all be considered, (Figure 20.4). The use of nutraceuticals in cats should be actively encouraged in the management of OA, as analgesia alternatives can be limited because there are few analgesia medications licensed for use in cats.

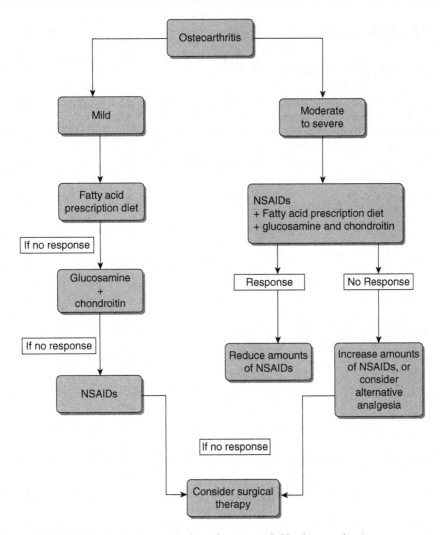

Figure 20.4   Flowchart of nutraceutical use in osteoarthritic dogs and cats.

Key points

- Maintain optimal weight.
- Increase the use of antioxidants in order to reduce the amount of free radicals.
- Encourage the use of nutraceuticals as a supplement or as part of dietary therapy.
- Ensure mobility is maintained, pain levels controlled, and quality of life is maintained.

References

Beale BS. Use of nutraceuticals and chondroprotectants in osteoarthritic dogs and cats. *Vet Clin North Am Small Anim Pract* 2004; 34(1):271–290.

May SA. Current research relevant to equine joint disease: Animal models and other experimental systems in the investigation of equine arthritis. In: McIlwraith CW, Trotter G, eds. *Joint Disease in the Horse*. Philadelphia: Saunders, 1996.

McIlwraith CW, Vachon A. Review of pathogenesis and treatment of degenerative joint disease. *Eq Vet J Suppl* 1998; 6:3–11.

21 Cancer

Nutrition can play an important role in the prevention and treatment of cancers. This does, however, vary with the type of tumour and stage of progression. The potential risk reduction of cancer when following dietary recommendations has not been well documented in veterinary medicine. In human studies 'eating right', staying active and maintaining a healthy weight can reduce the risk of cancer by 30–40% (Sheng-Long et al. 1992). It has been speculated that this reduction may be even more achievable in pets, as their dietary intake can be more controlled.

Cancer and nutrition

Correct feeding of the cancer patient can enhance quality and length of life. This is due to nutritional support reducing or preventing toxicoses associated with cancer therapy and ameliorating cancer-induced metabolic alterations. Anorexia is a common clinical symptom in cancer patients, which can lead to weight loss and cachexia in conjunction with the metabolic alterations. Use of body condition scores (BCS) can be an excellent monitoring tool to assess the overall nutritional effect of cancer and treatments.

Cancer affects the nutritional status of the animal in three ways:

- Therapy, e.g. chemotherapy-induced anorexia, nausea or vomiting. (Human chemotherapy patients have reported changes in taste and smell; these side effects experienced during therapy make it difficult for some patients to consume optimal quantity of calories and nutrients.)
- Alterations of the metabolic pathways
- Primary effect of tumours, such as compression or infiltration of the alimentary canal.

Cancer cachexia

Cachexia is defined as a profound and marked state of general ill health and malnutrition. It is a complex paraneoplastic syndrome including progressive weight

The Consulting Veterinary Nurse, First Edition. Nicola Ackerman.
© 2012 John Wiley & Sons, Ltd. Published 2012 by John Wiley & Sons, Ltd.

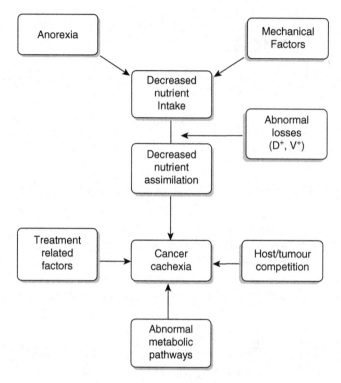

Figure 21.1 Factors that contribute to cancer cachexia.

loss that occurs despite adequate nutritional intake (Sheng-Long et al. 1992). Loss of both fat and muscle can occur, with the depletion of muscle mass often exceeding that of viscera in cancer patients. Cachexia is not very common in veterinary cancer patients, but weight loss usually occurs early in the course of the disease (Figure 21.1). Cachexia can cause a decreased quality of life, a decreased response to therapies and shortened survival time, when compared to those with similar diseases without cachexia. Cancer cachexia may be partly due to a negative energy balance. It is therefore important for the owner to have the animal weighed and BCS assessed on a regular basis.

Nurse clinics

The aims of nutritional management and of the nurse clinic are to:

- Provide an energy source for the patient that the tumour cannot readily utilise
- Meet the increased nutritional requirements of proteins
- Limit lactate production by the tumour
- Improve immune function, remission and survival times
- Aid in limiting tumour growth
- Perform repeat diagnostics

- Discuss compliance and medicating methods with owners, and answer any questions that the owners may have
- Provide further support to the client as required; some owners may wish to discuss euthanasia plans for the future.

Clinical nutrition

Carbohydrates

The metabolism of carbohydrates is greatly altered in dogs with cancer. The alteration in metabolism is due to tumours metabolising glucose via anaerobic glycolysis to lactic acid. A net energy gain by the tumour and net loss by the host results, as the host expends energy converting the lactate back to glucose. The alterations in metabolism are also suspected, but not yet proven, in cats. Hyperlactatemia can result, and this should be taken into consideration if intravenous fluid therapy is required. Hartmanns (lactated Ringer's) solution can exacerbate any hyperlactatemia and energy demands.

Carbohydrates can be poorly utilised as a result of peripheral insulin resistance; excess dietary soluble carbohydrates needs to be avoided. The nitrogen-free extract (NFE) value needs to be no more than 25% of dry matter or no more than 20% of metabolised energy. Providing metabolisable energy from fat is the most beneficial for the animal. Increased dietary fibre may aid in preventing abnormal stool quality (e.g. soft stools, or diarrhoea), which is commonly encountered when changing from a high-carbohydrate commercial dry food to a high-fat commercial or homemade diet. Recommendations of crude fibre levels greater than 2.5% on a dry matter basis (DMB) are documented (Sheng-Long et al. 1992).

Protein

Tumours use amino acids as a preferred source of energy. This results in an altered metabolism, with the patient having to increase skeletal protein breakdown, liver protein synthesis and whole body synthesis for tumour growth. This can become clinically significant when protein degradation exceeds intake. The immune response, wound healing rates and gastrointestinal functioning are also affected by the imbalances in protein levels. Specific amino acids are shown to have different effects in cancer patients.

Arginine and glutamine are commonly supplemented into diets specifically designed for cancer patients. The addition of arginine into total parenteral nutrition (TPN) solutions can decrease tumour growth and metabolic rate in rodent models. In canine models quality of life and survival time have been increased when dogs are fed arginine in conjunction with n-3 fatty acids. Glutamine is also added to most human and veterinary enteral formulas. Glutamine has shown to be beneficial in improving intestinal morphometry, reducing bacterial translocation, enhancing local immunity and improving survival times. Glutamine is a conditionally essential amino acid. Supplementation is recommended when protein metabolism is altered, as in cancer patients.

The amino acids methionine and asparagine are both used in tumour cell growth. Methionine's precursor, homocysteine, when supplemented to the diet can stop tumour cell growth progression into different growth phases. This enables cell-cycle specific therapeutic agents to target more tumour cells. Use of L-asparaginase in dogs and cats with lymphoma has high remission rates of 80%, because asparagine is an essential factor in cell growth. The supplementation of glycine can also have important implications depending on the type of chemotherapy being utilised. Glycine will reduce cisplatin-induced nephrotoxicity.

Fats

A larger proportion of the metabolisable energy should be from dietary fat and oils, because tumour cells have difficulty utilising fats and oils. If cachexia is present, an increase in dietary fat can improve the BCS. An ideal dietary fat content is 25–40% DMB, or 50–65% of the calories as an 'as fed' basis. Lipid metabolism also alters in cancer patients. Increased blood concentration of free fatty acids, very low-density lipoproteins, triglycerides, plasma lipoproteins and hormone-dependent lipoprotein lipase activity can occur due to an overall decrease in lipogenesis and increased lipolysis. These changes in lipid metabolism can also cause immunosuppression, which relates to a decrease in survival time.

Omega-3 (n-3) fatty acids, like EPA and DHA, generally have an inhibiting effect on tumour growth. EPA can decrease protein degradation without altering protein synthesis, thus aiding in the symptoms associated with cachexia. The ratio of omega-3 to omega-6 fatty acids is important, as omega-6 fatty acids such as linoleic and gamma-linolenic acid enhance metastases.

Vitamins and minerals

The levels of vitamins and minerals within the diet need to be sufficient to meet daily nutrient intakes. Higher levels of the antioxidant vitamins and minerals should be advocated in order to counteract damage caused by free radical action, and improve immune response (see Chapter 13). There are two hypotheses surrounding the use of antioxidants in cancer patients. The first supports the role of antioxidants within the diet as they may improve the efficacy of cancer therapy by improving immune function, increasing tumour response to radiation or chemotherapy, decreasing toxicity to normal cells and helping to reverse metabolic changes contributing towards cachexia (Roudebush et al. 2004). The second hypothesis states that antioxidants may have a deleterious effect by protecting cancer calls against damage by chemotherapy or radiation therapy (Roudebush et al. 2004).

Serum levels of the trace minerals zinc, chromium and iron are lower in dogs with lymphoma and osteosarcoma than in healthy dogs (Kazmierski et al. 2001). Diets that are complete and balanced should not need supplementation of these trace minerals, but in homemade diets it should be considered.

Feeding a cancer diet

Initial assessment of the patient needs to be performed. Regular reassessments and calculations of daily energy requirement (DER) will be required, especially if weight loss or cachexia starts to occur. If hospitalised, patients need to ingest at least their resting energy requirement (RER). At home, the calculated DER (RER × appropriate factor) is required. An initial illness factor of 1.25 in early stages of cancer increasing to 1.75 in later stages has been recommended, though illness factors should be used alongside daily weighing and BCS.

Because of the altered metabolism processes already discussed, modification of nutrient intake is required. Several veterinary therapeutic diets are available, and with an increased fat content are very palatable. A suitable period of transition on to the new diet is required. Some animals can suffer diarrhoea due to the increase in fat content, and may need a longer period of transition.

With all cancer patients care should be taken with monitoring weight loss, especially with those that are initially overweight. Rapid weight loss, due to anorexia and alterations in metabolism, can result in a loss of lean muscle mass. Fat stores may still remain and may mask the detrimental effect of protein catabolism. Careful muscle condition scores and BCS will need to be performed, as 'overcoat syndrome' can quite easily occur.

The use of appetite stimulants can be useful in some cancer patients. Diazepam or oxazepam are commonly used in practice, but can be unreliable in ensuring adequate calorie intake. Mirtazapine is a more widely used appetite stimulant (see Box 21.1).

Box 21.1   The use of mirtazapine as an appetite stimulant

Cats

- Dose rates 3.75 mg by mouth every 3 days, 25–50% dose reduction if renal failure was present
- In 31 cats, 26 (84%) of cats ate within 24 hours of administration of medication
- Of these 26, 100% continued to eat within 72 hours
- Two of the 31 (2%) cats showed side effects

Dogs

- Dose rates of 3.75 mg (<5 kg), 7.5 mg (5–10 kg), 11.25 mg (10–15 kg), 15 mg (15–30 kg), 22.75 mg (30–50 kg) and 30 mg (>50 kg), orally once daily
- Of 50 dogs, 43 (86%) ate within 24 hours
- Of these 43, 41(95%) continued to eat for 72 hours after administration of the first dose

Source: Casamian-Sorrosal and Warman (2010).

If appetite stimulants fail and long-term nutritional support is required, enteral feeding techniques will need to be considered. Active encouragement to eat still needs to be initiated by the owner, or by practice staff if the animal is hospitalised.

Support for the owner is especially required with cancer patients. The word cancer will make any owner anxious, especially if the animal is anorexic, which can be very distressing. Many animals will be sensitive to this in their owners, and this can be another factor associated with anorexia.

Key points

- Aim to prevent cancer cachexia.
- If the animal is unwilling to consume the cancer diet, inadequate calorific intake can result. It is best to feed anything, to ensure correct calorific intake.
- Quality of life for the animal is the most important factor.

References

Casamian-Sorrosal D, Warman S. The use of mirtazapine as an appetite stimulant in dogs and cats: a prospective observation study. *BSAVA Scientific Proceedings* 2010, p. 420.

Kazmierski KJ, Ogilvie GK, Fettman MJ, et al. Serum zinc, chromium and iron concentrations in dogs with lymphoma and osteosarcoma. *J Vet Intern Med* 2001; 15:585–588.

Roudebush P, Davenport DJ, Novotny BJ. The use of nutraceuticals in cancer therapy. *Vet Clin North Am Small Anim Pract* 2004; 34:249–269.

Sheng-Long YE, Istafan NW, Driscoll DF. Tumour and host response to arginine and branch chain amino acid enriched total parenteral nutrition. *Cancer* 1992; 69:261–270.

22 Cardiac Disorders

The nutritional status of the cardiac patient is exceptionally important to ascertain, as it can have several effects on the animal. These can include the choice and dose rate of the drugs used in the medical treatment, interpretation of any laboratory results, interpretation of ECG data, prognosis of both surgical and medical intervention, and the choice of diet for the patient. As part of the initial clinical assessment, a full history of the animal's diet should be taken (Appendix 1). Nutrition can be a causative factor in cardiac disease. If the animal receives unusual supplements or is not fed a complete diet, if more than one animal in the household is affected or if it is being fed a homemade or fad diet, cardiac disease can be induced. Micro- and macronutrient deficiencies (calcium, potassium) can cause cardiac problems and thus a complete blood work-up is necessary.

Assessment of the animal's body condition and muscle scores (BCS and MCS) is important with cardiac patients. A reduction in skeletal muscle mass might indicate energy malnutrition, and possibly a negative nitrogen balance. Animals with catabolic disease, such as hyperthyroidism and cardiac failure lose body mass very rapidly, as with anorexic cats. The progression of cardiac disease can be exacerbated in obese animals. This can result in cardiomegaly, circulatory congestion, oedema, ascites and hypocalcaemia. An overweight animal must be subjectively assessed; obesity must be differentiated from abdominal distension due to hepatomegaly or ascites. Obesity can also mask an underlying lean muscle body mass. Radiography can be useful in determining lack of lean body mass; this is especially noticeable on the proximal limbs. Obese animals need to lose weight in a controlled, monitored way, the same as in a normal healthy animal. Obesity not only produces clinical signs (see Table 22.1) that mimic those of early heart failure, but can also cause cardiovascular changes that can exacerbate any underlying cardiovascular disease (see Box 22.1).

The Consulting Veterinary Nurse, First Edition. Nicola Ackerman.
© 2012 John Wiley & Sons, Ltd. Published 2012 by John Wiley & Sons, Ltd.

Table 22.1 Functional classification of heart failure and corresponding sodium intake

Class	Description[a]	Recommended upper limits of sodium intake (mg/kg body weight per day)
I	Normal physical activity: symptoms not induced under normal exercise levels	Unrestricted
II	Slightly limited physical capacity: original physical activity leads to clinical signs	6.8
III	Markedly limited physical capacity: limited physical activity leads to clinical signs	4.5
IV	Unable to carry on any activity without signs: clinical signs present at rest	2.8

[a]Clinical signs include weight loss, exercise intolerance, coughing, respiratory distress and occasionally ascites.

Box 22.1 Cardiovascular adaptations that occur during the transition from ideal BCS to obesity

- Increased perfusion requirements of expanding adipose tissue
- Elevated cardiac output
- Abnormal left ventricular function
- Variable blood pressure response (normotensive to hypertensive)
- Increased retention of sodium and water by the kidney
- Increased plasma aldosterone and noradrenaline (norepinephrine) concentration
- Increase left arterial pressure
- Increased heart rate
- Exercise intolerance

Nurse clinics

The aims of nursing clinics and clinical nutrition in cardiac disease are to:

- Help control signs associated with sodium and fluid retention, by avoiding nutritional deficiencies and excesses
- Aid in maintaining normal heart muscle function
- Slow the progression of any concurrent renal disease
- Support patients receiving diuretics or angiotensin converting enzyme (ACE) inhibitors, aiding the client with compliance in administration of medications
- Maintain optimal weight and body condition score to aid in preventing cardiac cachexia
- Monitor blood pressure and other diagnostic signs
- Provide support to the owner, as and when required.

Cardiac cachexia

A large proportion (34–75%) of dogs with heart disease suffer from anorexia, and is it one of the multifactorial processes associated with the loss of lean body mass in cardiac cachexia (Freeman and Rush 2005). Other factors include increased energy requirements and metabolic alterations. Cardiac cachexia is more commonly seen in dogs than in cats, and in dilated cardiomyopathy (DCM) or right-sided heart failure.

The primary energy source for animals with acute or chronic disease is amino acids from muscle, thus causing a reduction in lean body mass. Cachexia is a slow, progressive process of the loss of lean body mass/muscle. Obese animals should be examined carefully, as this lean body mass reduction can cause 'overcoat syndrome' (see Chapter 10), and thus be easily missed. The clinical nutrition of these animals includes management of any anorexia present.

Clinical nutrition

L-Carnitine

L-Carnitine is critical for fatty acid metabolism and energy production, and cardiac myocytes depend on the oxidation of fatty acids for their energy. A causative link between L-carnitine deficiencies and DCM has not been established, although L-carnitine deficiencies within the cardiac myocytes occur in 50% of dogs with DCM. Some dogs with DCM respond to L-carnitine supplementation. Supplementation of 50–100 mg/kg body weight orally every 8 hours has been recommended to for with DCM, although most cardiac diets are already supplemented with L-carnitine (Freeman and Rush 2005).

Fats

The role of fatty acids in the diet of cardiac patients has been widely reported. Supplementation of the diet with eicosapentaenoic acid (EPA) and docosahexaenoic acid (DHA) has been shown to improve cachexia scores, but had no effect on survival time, thus improving quality of life. Animals suffering from cardiac cachexia have an increased production of inflammatory cytokines. These cytokines are directly linked to anorexia, increasing energy requirements and catabolism of lean body mass (Freeman and Rush 2005). Supplementation of the diet with omega-3 fatty acids (especially EPA and DHA) decreases the production and effects of cytokines.

Recommended dosage of 40 mg/kg body weight of EPA and 25 mg/kg body weight of DHA for both dogs and cats with anorexia or cachexia have been noted (Freeman and Rush 2005). With most fish oil supplements containing 180 mg EPA and 120 mg of DHA per capsule, dosages can be easily calculated (Freeman and Rush 2005). Specific fatty acid supplements are now available for cardiac patients.

Carbohydrates

The level of carbohydrates in the diet has to provide adequate calories for the animal's life stage. In most cases of cardiac disease this is for senior animals, so the required calorific value of the diet tends to be lower. It should also be remembered that these animals tend to have a more sedentary lifestyle due to their cardiac disease, and the risk for weight gain, or already being obese, is greater.

The recommended level of fibre in the diet is very much dependent on the individual. For an obese animal, it is initially recommended that the animal reduces in weight, to reach its optimal body weight and BCS. This may involve the use of a high-fibre diet. In animals which are already at an ideal BCS and optimal weight, fibre should be present but not excessive. The presence of fibre in the diet reduces the bioavailability of many of the nutrients. As concurrent disease or impairment of the gastrointestinal tract, pancreas and liver can occur in cardiac patients, a high-fibre diet may not be ideal (Roudebush 2000).

Vitamins and minerals

The nutrients of main concern in patients with heart failure include sodium, potassium and magnesium. The treats and snacks that are often fed to dogs have a high salt content, as do cheese and processed meats, which are often used to help administer medications. The restriction of sodium in the diet is useful as it helps to reduce the fluid retention that accompanies many forms of heart disease (see Table 22.1). Both sodium and water can be retained when the renin–angiotensin–aldosterone (RAA) cascade is stimulated, or when the patient's blood pressure falls (Davies 1996).

One of the current methods of treatment for fluid retention is the use of diuretics. The diuretics block sodium retention but also promote urinary loss of magnesium and potassium. The prolonged use of diuretics can also lead to deficiencies of the water-soluble vitamins. Stimulation of the RAA cascade results in an increase of extracellular and vascular fluid volume, thus increasing preload. The plasma protein concentration therefore becomes more dilute, which in turn decreases plasma oncotic pressure. Water moves from the vascular to the interstitial compartment, resulting in oedema, ascites and congestion.

The use of ACE inhibitors has led to modification of the recommendation for sodium restriction in senior diets and early cardiac disease diets. ACE inhibitors are designed to block the production of angiotensin II and its subsequent stimulation of the secretion of aldosterone. Both of these chemicals promote retention of water and sodium by the kidney. Thus ACE inhibitors result in impaired sodium and water excretion. Sodium intake needs to be limited in proportion to the severity of the disease (see Table 22.1), in an attempt to avoid excesses. ACE inhibitors can also cause potassium retention, thus periodic serum levels should be monitored (Buffington et al. 2004). Spironolactone has similar potassium-sparing effects, along with being an aldosterone antagonist.

Chronic renal failure (CRF) is often a concomitant disease of patients with cardiovascular disorders. Diets for these animals also need restricted phosphorus levels. Levels of potassium and magnesium should also optimally controlled, as this supports the patient receiving diuretics and/or ACE inhibitor therapy.

Magnesium levels can have a deleterious effect on a range of cardiovascular conditions including hypertension, congestive heart failure (CHF), coronary artery disease and cardiac arrhythmias (Buffington et al. 2004). Hypomagnesaemia can be induced through the use of digoxin and loop diuretics.

The B vitamin complexes are often supplemented into cardiac diets. At yet there has been little investigation into the role of vitamin B deficiency as a cause of heart disease in dogs and cats. Polyuria and anorexia can both contribute to low vitamin B concentrations, and thus B vitamin requirements are higher.

Recommendations for higher levels of antioxidants in animals suffering from CHF are commonplace, due to the by-products of reactive oxygen species (ROS). The antioxidant coenzyme Q_{10} has been anecdotally recommended; like L-carnitine, it is a cofactor in a number of energy-producing reactions. Benefits of supplementation include improved myocardial metabolic efficiency and increases in antioxidant production (Freeman and Rush 2005). Although no hard evidence has established the direct benefits of coenzyme Q_{10}, dosages of 30 mg orally twice a day, and in large breeds of dogs up to 90 mg orally twice a day, are thought to be beneficial (Freeman and Rush 2005).

Proteins

Taurine is an essential amino acid in cats, because in feline metabolism it is the only amino acid able to combine with cholesterol during bile salt synthesis, whereas in other species another amino acid, glycine, can be substituted. Cats have a limited ability to synthesise taurine from cysteine and methionine, but its use outstrips production. The mechanism of heart failure in cats and dogs with taurine deficiency is poorly understood. Until 1987 the supplementation of commercial foods with taurine was not commonplace and the number of cases of feline DCM was large.

Clinical studies have also shown that inadequate potassium intake may be sufficient to induce a significant taurine depletion and cardiovascular disease in cats. Most dogs presenting with DCM do not tend to have a concurrent taurine deficiency, but a taurine deficiency has been noted in some breeds where DCM is not a common disease. Dog breeds reported to be associated with taurine deficiency include American cocker spaniel, golden retriever, Labrador, Newfoundland, Dalmatian and English bulldog (Freeman and Rush 2005).

The overall protein level is reduced in cardiac diets. This is due to the progression of renal disease, which is associated with cardiac disease. The protein levels are therefore restricted but of a high biological value: typical values of 17% (DMB) for dogs and 29% (DMB) for cats are often recommended.

It should be noted that if protein restriction is too great this can be detrimental to the animal. Protein malnutrition can rapidly occur in the presence of catabolic disease and inadequate food intake. Hypoproteinaemia can be present in cardiac disease with reduced liver function. In animals with cardiac cachexia, protein levels should be increased. Supplementing a cardiac diet with scrambled eggs or cottage cheese is an excellent method of increasing the protein levels without increasing the salt content of the diet.

Feeding the cardiac patient

Each diet must be based on the individual's specific requirements. Overweight or obese animals will require diets aimed at restricting calories, underweight patients a calorie-dense diet. Concurrent disease also needs to be taken into consideration. Laboratory parameters should be obtained to identify any electrolyte excesses or deficiencies. Anorexia is a common side effect of CHF, and the owner may have to make great efforts in order to entice the animal to eat.

Feeding a low-salt diet

Low-salt diets are used for both cardiac and renal patients. It is often a misconception that low-salt diets have a reduced palatability. Studies have demonstrated that diets with reduced sodium chloride levels used in patients with cardiovascular or renal disease have palatability comparable to that of supermarket brands, or better (see Table 22.2) (Roudebush et al. 2000).

Difficulties in transition from the patient's original diet to a low-salt prescription diet can be attributed to:

- Advanced illness associated with renal and heart failure
- Established eating and feeding habits of both the animal and the owner
- Anorexia associated with disease process and/or medications
- Too quick a transition and/or established food aversions.

Table 22.2 Comparison of feeding restricted sodium diets vs commercial diets with a high comparison sodium level

Food A	Food B	Preferring Food A (%)	Preferring Food B (%)	Number of animals
Canine h/d[a], dry	Purina Dog Chow	95	5	60
Canine h/d, dry	Iams Chunks	60	40	60
Canine h/d, dry	Pedigree Chum original	95	5	60
Canine h/d, canned	Ken-L-Ration Original	100	0	60

[a]Hill's Prescription Diet Canine h/d.

Table 22.3 Daily sodium intake for a dog and cat eating various foods; based on a 15 kg dog consuming 935 kcal/day, and a 4 kg cat consuming 270 kcal/day

Food	Sodium intake (mg/day)
Dog	
Grocery moist diet	2845
Grocery dry diet	1144
Senior dry diet	390
Renal moist diet	400
Cardiac dry diet	111
30 g cheese	262
1 slice of bread	218
Cat	
Grocery moist diet	952
Grocery dry food	371
Senior dry diet	186
Renal/cardiac moist diet	175
Renal/cardiac dry diet	156
½ tin tuna	160

Transition to a low-salt diet is always easier if the animal has already been fed a diet in a lower salt category. Animals are often encouraged to consume a new diet by adding flavour enhancers. Low-sodium additives can include low-sodium soups and sweeteners, such as honey or syrups. Table 22.3 demonstrates how adding certain foodstuffs to the diet can significantly increase the sodium intake.

As with all clinical prescription diets, the therapeutic agent of the diet should not be imposed if it is detrimental to the overall nutrient intake. Owners should be aware that a process of trial and error may be required for these patients. Some animals can 'go off' certain diets, and a cyclical approach with two or three commercial prescription diets may be required. Different feeding methods along with different foods should be tried. The success of a transition of a new diet depends hugely on the dedication of the owner and the support received from the veterinary practice. One way in which the owner can be supported by providing a list of foodstuffs and their sodium content. If the animal is overweight or underweight then a weight management programme must be initiated.

Administering medications can be difficult, and many of the foods used to 'hide' them can be high in salt. Advising owners on different methods can lead to an increase in compliance. Alternatives can include:

- Teaching the owner to administer medications without the use of foods, which can include the use of pill givers
- The use of commercial treats designed to hold medications (but always double-check the salt content)
- Use of appropriate foods such as bananas (good potassium source), no-added-salt peanut butter (not ideal in obese animals), and home-cooked meats (without added salt), not sandwich/processed meats.

Key points

- Ensure that the daily calorie and nutrient intake is met.
- The optimal BCS needs to be achieved in both obese and underweight animals.

References

Buffington T, Holloway C, Abood S. *Manual of Veterinary Dietetics*. St Louis, MO: Elsevier Saunders, 2004.

Davies M. Feeding the cardiac patient. In: Kelly N, Wills J, eds. *BSAVA Manual of Companion Animal Nutrition and Feeding*. Gloucester: BSAVA Publications, 1996, pp. 117–127.

Freeman LM, Rush JE. Nutritional modulation of heart disease In: Ettinger SJ, Feldman EC, eds. *Textbook of Veterinary Internal Medicine*, volume 1, 6th edition. St Louis, MO: Elsevier Saunders, 2005.

Roudebush P. Study cited in Roudebush P, Keene BW, Mizelle L. Cardiovascular disease. In: Hand MS, Thatcher CD, Remillard RL, Roudebush P, eds. *Small Animal Clinical Nutrition*, 4th edition. Topeka, KS: Mark Morris Institute, 2000, pp. 529–562.

Roudebush P, Keene BW, Mizelle L. Cardiovascular Disease. In: Hand MS, Thatcher CD, Remillard RL, Roudebush P, eds. *Small Animal Clinical Nutrition*, 4th edition. Topeka, KS: Mark Morris Institute, 2000, pp. 529–562.

23 Cognitive Dysfunction

'Cognitive dysfunction' is a term used to describe geriatric behavioural changes that are not solely attributable to a general medical condition, such as infection, organ failure or neoplasm (Frank 2000). Other terms such as 'senile dementia' and 'senile degeneration of the brain' are also often used. It should be remembered that cognitive dysfunction should not be considered as a normal part of the ageing process. It is, rather, a pathological condition that can result from encephalitis, tumours or other structural diseases, metabolic conditions (e.g. hypothyroidism), or an idiopathic cause.

Nurse clinics

The aims of the nursing clinic for pets suffering from cognitive dysfunction are to:

- Help to reduce the behavioural changes associated with cognitive dysfunction
- Feed a nutritionally balanced diet, aimed at the senior life stage
- Reduce oxidative stress by neutralising free radicals, and thus preventing extensive cellular damage
- Aid the client in coping with behavioural changes the animal may show

Clinical nutrition

Proteins

The protein levels in diets aimed at animals with cognitive dysfunction need to be similar to those in senior life stage diets. Levels tend to be around 19–20% (DMB). This is to help maintain heart and kidney health in the senior animal.

The Consulting Veterinary Nurse, First Edition. Nicola Ackerman.
© 2012 John Wiley & Sons, Ltd. Published 2012 by John Wiley & Sons, Ltd.

Carbohydrates

The levels of carbohydrates within the diet need to reflect that senior animals can be less active than younger adults. The calorific level of the carbohydrate content can therefore be decreased, but it is recommended though that the fibre content of senior diets should be higher than that of adult life stage diets. Bowel function in older dogs can be decreased, and the addition of fibre can assist in its functioning. Carbohydrate (NFE) levels are recommended to be around 55% (DMB), and crude fibre at 4.5% (DMB).

Fats

The overall level of fats within the diet also needs to reflect that of a senior diet. The type of fats contained within the diet is important. Levels of the omega-3 (n-3) fatty acids DHA and EPA need to be increased. These fats contribute to neuronal cell membrane plasticity and health (Youdim et al. 2000). The decline in structural and functional integrity of the brain tissue correlates with the loss of DHA concentrations from the cell membranes. The brain is rich in polyunsaturated fatty acids (PUFAs), especially DHA, with concentrations of PUFAs directly reflecting concentrations within the diet. It has therefore been concluded that diets with increased levels of omega-6 and omega-3 fatty acids may help to delay or reduce the onset of neurodegenerative disorders such as cognitive dysfunction (Youdim et al. 2000).

A natural phospholipid, phosphatidylserine, has been added to some supplements designed to aid in cognitive dysfunction. The main physiological effect is to enhance and maintain the cell activities based on the functionality of the plasma membrane.

Vitamins and minerals

The levels of the vitamins and minerals that act as antioxidants are increased in diets intended for dogs with cognitive dysfunction, because the antioxidants help to protect against free radical damage. The main antioxidants used are vitamins E and C, beta-carotene and selenium. Vitamin E is used to help neutralise free radical reactivity. Antioxidants are believed to promote recovery in neurons that are exhibiting signs of neuropathology and therefore nutritional manipulation is believed to offer useful medication-related treatments for cognitive dysfunction. Vitamin C regenerates vitamin E, restoring its antioxidant activity. Beta-carotene reinforces vitamin E and also boosts its antioxidant capacity. Selenium in the diet aids by being a component of the antioxidant enzyme glutathione peroxidase.

The levels of other vitamins and minerals within the diet need to reflect levels required by animals at a senior life stage.

Feeding a dog with cognitive dysfunction

Diets have been designed to encompass all of these nutritional components. The difficulty arises when the animal is suffering from another disease or disorder, and requires a diet specifically for this problem. Supplements have been designed that contain the antioxidants recommended for cognitive dysfunction. The levels of fatty acids are more difficult to increase, but this can be achieved by using oil supplements.

As diets aimed at cognitive dysfunction are based around a senior life stage diet, few side effects are experienced when changing. However, it should be remembered that older dogs can be fussier with their diets and transition to a new diet can be difficult. Owners should also be advised that there is no cure for cognitive dysfunction, only help in delaying some of the symptoms. Regular examinations at the veterinary practice should be advocated, along with medications if required.

Key points

- Feed depending on the animal's body condition score (BCS) and weight. Specific cognitive dysfunction diets are aimed at animals with an ideal weight and BCS
- Supplements can be used if the animal is on a specific diet for a concurrent condition
- Cognitive dysfunction is not an inevitable consequence of old age.

References

Frank D. Cognitive Dysfunction in dogs. *Hill's European Symposium on Canine Brain Ageing* 2000. pp. 22–27.

Youdim KA, Martin A and Joseph JA. Essential fatty acids and the brain: possible health implications. *Int J Dev Neurosci* 2000; 18:383–399.

24 Dental Problems

Dental disease is the most common problem suffered by adult dogs and cats. The incidence rates for some form of dental disease are as much as 85% in dogs and 70% in cats over the age of 3 (Stiefel et al. 1992). The development of periodontal disease is dependent on the host's immunity and inflammatory responses to plaque on the tooth surface (Furniss 2006).

Dental disease is preventable, and many clinics are devoted to educating clients how to prevent dental disease by tooth brushing or diet. The nurse's role in preventive health care is easily demonstrated in dental care. Puppies and kittens that are habituated to having their mouths handled and their teeth brushed are at an advantage with their dental hygiene. All puppy and kitten owners should have instructions on how to perform these tasks.

Nurse clinics

The aim of nursing dentistry clinics are to:

- Encourage chewing: this can be achieved by using kibbles of different sizes
- Limit the components of plaque, and the mineralisation of plaque to tartar
- Increase antimicrobial action, with the use of chlorohexidine products
- Encourage the owner to habituate the animal to having its mouth handled and its teeth examined
- Teach the owner how to achieve effective toothbrushing
- Identify when other methods such as ultrasonic descaling are required.

As previously mentioned, all owners puppies and kittens should have toothbrushing demonstrated to them and actively encouraged during puppy and kitten clinics. Owners of older animals should also be encouraged to brush their pet's teeth, through nurse clinics. An ideal time for referral is from annual vaccinations. All animals that have had some form of dental procedure should be referred to nurse clinics. Those that have only received dental hygiene treatment should see

The Consulting Veterinary Nurse, First Edition. Nicola Ackerman.
© 2012 John Wiley & Sons, Ltd. Published 2012 by John Wiley & Sons, Ltd.

the veterinary nurse about 3 days after the procedure for guidance on ongoing homecare. Those that have had extractions or have severe gingivitis should initially see a veterinary surgeon after the procedure. Once the veterinary surgeon is happy, the client should be referred to the veterinary nurse for homecare advice. All post-procedure protocols are very much dependent on the practice's general protocols and each individual patient. Owners should be encouraged to use a chlorohexidine-based product, rather than an enzymatic paste, for all animals that have received dental treatment.

Follow-up appointments should be as required, with a minimum of 3 months between check-ups with the clinic. Disclosing swabs or fluids and specific ultra violet lights can be very helpful in identifying areas of the teeth that the owner needs to concentrate on, and the effectiveness of the overall homecare being used. Many insurance companies now require routine dental hygiene checks, at least two or three a year, before they will provide cover for dental procedures.

Toothbrushing

Toothbrushing is the gold standard in oral hygiene care. Young animals should be habituated to having their heads, and then their mouths, handled. The use of flavoured tooth pastes can facilitate this process. Many clients have difficulty with the pet trying to consume the paste. Pushing the gel or paste well into the bristles of the brush can prevent the pet from eating the paste before it reaches the teeth.

Enzymatic toothpastes are ideal in healthy mouths of breeds of dogs not predisposed to dental disease. As periodontal disease can start in predisposed breeds from a very young age, it is recommended that a chlorohexidine-based paste or gel is used in these animals from an early age, i.e. puppyhood. The staining that this product can cause can easily be removed with brushing, and cosmetically is not a problem in animals as it is with people.

Instructing clients on how to start toothbrushing with their pet is important. The length of time it takes to reach full brushing will depend on the pet, and the proficiency of the owner. The length of each step is dependent on many factors and, as the person giving guidance, you should use common sense depending on how quickly the owner progresses through the following stages:

1   Handling the pet's head and mouth
2   Habituating the pet to having a gel or paste applied around its gums
3   Moving on to gently brushing the teeth with a small-headed toothbrush.

The actual brushing of the teeth and gums should be done with a medium-grade brush. Small-headed brushes are ideal for starting owners off with brushing. Finger brushes tend to be too bulky in the mouth, with the rubber 'bristles' too big to perform adequate subgingival brushing. The mouth should always be kept closed during brushing as the lingual aspect of the teeth rarely requires brushing. The front of the mouth is the most sensitive part, as it is the area that would 'feel' what the animal is eating, shearing off pieces of food. The rear of the mouth is less sensitive, as it concentrates on the chewing of the food. It can therefore be more difficult to brush the front of the animal's mouth than the rear.

Some gingival bleeding is to be expected when initiating toothbrushing, as the gums are not accustomed to the abrasive nature of brushing. This will normally pass in a few days; however, if it does continue, this can indicate gingivitis, and guidance from a veterinary surgeon should be sought.

If you advocate the use of finger brushes and other materials such as flannels or swabs to apply gels and pastes, it should be remembered that the animal in question may not be totally comfortable with toothbrushing and there is a potential that it may bite. As the owner's fingers are in the animal's mouth, the owner should be warned about the potential for biting. If at any point you feel that the animal could have the potential to bite the owner, whether with intent or not, different forms of dental hygiene should be advocated; for example dental diets, oral rinse and drinking-water additives.

Chlorohexidine products

Chlorohexidine is an ideal disinfectant for use in oral hygiene, and is readily available in many forms and different concentrations. Oral rinses can be used in animals that owners find difficult to brush, either because of the pet's behaviour or the owner's inability to brush the teeth. Gels are highly palatable and can be wiped into the animal's mouth or even placed onto the back of a cat's paw, so that they can be licked off. In a study conducted in severely disabled people chlorhexidine gel was compared with placebo. Swabbing with chlorhexidine resulted in consistent, and, in part, significant improvements in plaque, gingivitis and periodontal pocket depth. Side effects of chlorhexidine (i.e. tooth stain and calculus) were relatively minor. Perceived improvements in dental health were associated with improved physical health, appearance and mouth odour. The results indicate that chlorhexidine swabbing is a useful oral disease preventive protocol for people with disabilities, and extrapolations can be made to the veterinary field (Stiefel et al. 1992). This study therefore indicates that chlorhexidine is a useful tool in the treatment and prevention of periodontal disease in animals where brushing cannot be performed.

Drinking-water additives

Additives can be added in the animal's drinking-water that can help in formation of plaque. Xylitol is the active ingredient, and in the quantities found in these additives it has beneficial effects.

Xylitol is a naturally occurring sugar substitute derived from plants and is found in many human 'sugar-free' products, such as gum and other sweets. In humans, high doses may have a mild laxative effect, but in dogs the ingestion of a high dose could be fatal. There is a link between xylitol ingestion and hypoglycaemia in dogs, as xylitol can cause an increase in insulin secretion. Diabetic chocolate contains two toxic ingredients, as it contains large amounts of xylitol as well as the theobromine in the chocolate. Other symptoms of xylitol overdose include vomiting, weakness, ataxia, depression, hypokalaemia, seizures, coma and liver dysfunction and/or failure. Some clients will naturally have questions about the addition of xylitol to their pet's water bowl, but it is perfectly safe in small quantities, and beneficial to dental health.

Diet

The diet of the animal can play an important preventive and therapeutic role. The type of food consumed, its texture and composition directly affect the oral environment. The use of dental diets and their overall effectiveness depends on three factors:

- The level of plaque present on the teeth, and the animal's response to the plaque on the teeth (gingivitis)
- The owner's ability to accomplish dental homecare on the pet (e.g. toothbrushing)
- The selection of the methods of oral homecare by the veterinary practice for the owner. Consideration should include products that are most likely to ensure compliance; this also includes the cost of the products.

Dental diets are designed with a few different mechanisms. The kibble size is influential: large kibbles force the animal to chew the kibble, increasing chewing activity. The texture of the diet, especially if it is high in fibre, has been shown to be beneficial in the removal of plaque and calculus from the teeth (Figure 24.1). Calculus is formed by the mineralisation of plaque, particularly by calcium.

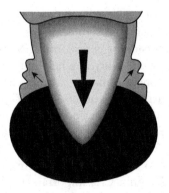

Figure 24.1 Diagram demonstrating how fibre alignment within the kibble can wipe the tooth surface of plaque.

Calcium is secreted in the saliva, and this explains why teeth located next to salivary ducts tend to have larger calcium deposits than other teeth. The use of polyphosphates in the diet is to bind the calcium from the saliva, making it unavailable for the formation of calculus. The calcium is then released as normal in the digestive tract and absorbed by the animal. The use of polyphosphates is more effective as a coating on the kibble rather than incorporated into the kibble (Furniss 2006).

Clinical nutrition

Carbohydrates

The use of fibre in the kibble is proven to reduce plaque and calculus formation accumulating on the tooth. High levels of other forms of carbohydrate can be detrimental. Plaque bacteria use fermentable carbohydrates, such as glucose, as a source of energy. The by-products of this process are acidic and cause demineralisation of the enamel, allowing caries to form (Tutt 2006). Changes in the diet along with dental homecare can prevent the formation of caries in dogs. Caries in cats is exceptionally rare, but has been reported (Tutt 2006).

Protein

A diet deficient in protein has shown to cause degenerative changes in the periodontium. As protein deficiencies rarely occur in dogs and cats, in practice this is not a typical cause of periodontal disease. In some diets, protein levels are moderately reduced in order to limit the components of plaque.

Vitamins and minerals

Calcium and phosphorus consumed in unbalanced ratios can lead to secondary nutritional hyperparathyroidism and significant loss of alveolar bone. The loss of bone can support the progression of periodontitis. Moderately reducing the levels of calcium in the diet, or its availability, can help limit the mineralisation of plaque to tartar. The addition of polyphosphates (calcium-chelating agents) can produce a significant reduction in tartar formation (~45%) (Gorrel and Derbyshire 2005). Zinc has both antibacterial and healing properties, and promotes a healthy epithelium (Servet et al. 2003). Zinc salts can also inhibit the formation of tartar (calculus) (Dethioux et al. 2005).

Vitamins C and A can also aid in dental problems, and are sometimes supplemented into dental diets. Vitamin C is important in the production of collagen, which is the main protein found within the gums. Vitamin A aids in protecting the epithelium.

Feeding a dental diet

The use of dental diets is aimed primarily at preventing and removing small amounts of plaque and calculus. If the animal has larger amounts of calculus or periodontal disease, dental descaling and polishing will be required. Prophylactic diets, chews and toothbrushing can be recommended after dentistry. Most diets designed for dentistry are based around a senior life stage diet, and animals that require a diet with a high energy density may require addition calories from another source. Dental diets are poor at removing plaque from the subgingival area, and dental hygiene procedures (toothbrushing) will be required to remove this debris.

Dental hygiene chews are widely used, mainly due to the ease of compliance. Owners love the idea that they are giving their pet a treat that is also a preventive treatment, but guidance needs to be followed with the use of these dental chews. Chews are often based on a rice flour formula and have a calorific value. Manufacturer's guidelines state that a portion of the daily food ration needs to be removed if a chew is given. Rawhide-based chews have limited calorific value, but the chew should be removed when it becomes small enough for the dog to attempt to swallow it. Choking can easily occur at this stage, and supervision of the dog is recommended.

Key points

- Prevalence of dental disease in dogs, cats and rabbits is exceptionally high and so nurse clinics should include both prevention and management strategies.
- Nurses should have a wide range of dental products available (Figure 24.2), so that clients have options for different methods of dental hygiene.

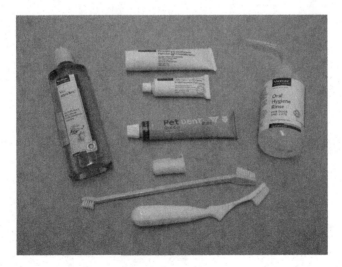

Figure 24.2 Examples of dental hygiene products.

- When instigating toothbrushing, be prepared to build up in stages and ensure that the pet is completely happy with each stage before moving on to the next.

References

Dethioux F, Marniquet P, Petit P, Weber M. How can we combat mouth disorders? *Focus Special Edition: Preventative nutrition for major health risks in cats* 2005, pp. 29–36.

Furniss G. The role of nutrition in the dental care of dogs and cats. *Vet Rev* 2006; 114:50–54.

Gorrel C, Derbyshire S. *Veterinary Dentistry for the Nurse and Technician*. Oxford: Elsevier Butterworth Heinemann, 2005.

Servet E, Hendriks W, Clarke D. Taking care of cats' teeth – kibbles can be useful in the prevention of periodontal disease. *Waltham Focus* 2003; 13(3):32–35.

Stiefel DJ, Truelove EL, Chin MM, Mandel LS. Efficacy of chlorhexidine swabbing in oral health care for people with severe disabilities. *Spec Care Dentist* 1992; 12:57–62.

Tutt C. Tooth friendly diets. *UK Vet* 2006; 11(6):78–80.

25 Diabetes

Diabetes mellitus is a complex disease, with stabilisation of blood glucose levels being affected by confounding disease processes, efficacy of the primary disease control treatment, diet and exercise programme, and weight control. Thus a full history of the animal, including all these factors, must be taken.

There are several possible causes of diabetes mellitus, including pancreatitis, obesity, drugs (glucocorticoids, progestins), concurrent illness (hyperadrenocorticism, acromegaly), genetics, immune-mediated insulitis, infections and islet amyloidosis. Obtaining an ideal body condition score (BCS) in both cats and dogs is the end goal in all of these cases, with obesity increasing the risk of diabetes in cats fourfold. Obese diabetic animals may have difficulty losing weight, but stabilisation of the diabetes is the initial aim, followed by a conservative weight loss programme, which needs to be carefully monitored by a veterinary professional.

Underweight animals, once stabilised, should be fed a modest increase in calories in order to promote repletion. Dietary therapy can only help to improve glycaemic control, but emphasis should be placed on adjustment of the dosage and schedule of insulin (or oral hypoglycemic, although these are not commonly used, as they are not very efficacious), and control of concurrent disease (Michel 2005).

In insulin-dependent diabetes (IDDM or type 1 diabetes), the beta cells of the pancreas lose their ability to secrete insulin (Stogdale 1986). This can be congenital or as a result of pancreatitis, or prolonged disease to the pancreas. Exogenous insulin administration is required as the treatment. The monitoring of pancreatic specific enzymes should also occur when conducting routine monitoring of these cases, as it can be a primary cause.

Type 2 diabetes (NIDDM) is defined as insulin resistance occurring at the site of the peripheral tissues. Dysfunction of the beta cells can also be a causal factor (Figure 25.1). The quantity of insulin secreted by the beta cells may be increased or decreased, or may remain normal. In some texts type 2 diabetes that resolves is sometimes classed as transient type 2. This is more commonly seen in obese cats when insulin resistance becomes established. Once the cat attains and then maintains an ideal BCS, type 2 diabetes can resolve itself. If the beta cells become

The Consulting Veterinary Nurse, First Edition. Nicola Ackerman.
© 2012 John Wiley & Sons, Ltd. Published 2012 by John Wiley & Sons, Ltd.

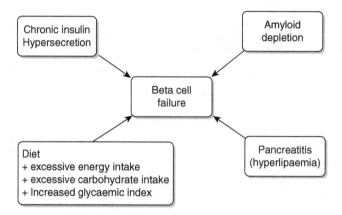

Figure 25.1 Physiopathology of insulin-resistant diabetes.

exhausted, a period of exogenous insulin administration may be required. The beta cells can start secreting insulin again after a period of time, and therefore this is not a true type 2 diabetes.

Hyperglycaemia is toxic to beta cells and aggravates the situation by further reducing insulin secretion. This mechanism can also explain why the more obese the animal, and the longer the animal has been obese, the greater the incidence of the onset of diabetes. There are many factors that can predispose the animal to insulin resistance (see Box 25.1).

Box 25.1   Factors that can predispose to insulin resistance

- Obesity
- Hyperadrenocorticism (HAC/Cushing's disease)
- Dioestrus
- Diabetogenic medications
- Acromegaly
- Infections (e.g. dental or urinary)
- Hyper- and hypothyroidism
- Chronic renal failure
- Congestive hepatic failure
- Congestive cardiac failure
- Hyperlipidaemia
- Hypercalcaemia
- Pancreatitis
- Neoplasm

Nurse clinics

The involvement of the nurse in diabetic cases is very important, and plays a major role in the overall health of the patient. The concept of diabetes and the necessary management regimes can be very overwhelming for some pet owners. There is a lot of information for people to take in, and having a series of clinics can be very beneficial. When lots of information needs to be disseminated, the use of handouts and recommended websites can be very helpful.

The aims of nursing clinics for diabetic cases are to:

- Ensure that the owners are happy with their understanding of diabetes, and what and why the different aspects of diabetes management will help their pet
- Ensure that the owners are competent in the administering of the correct quantity of insulin, identification of hypoglycaemic episodes, storage of insulin, requirements for repetitive blood tests, e.g. glucose curves and fructosamine levels
- Aid in compliance and act as point of contact for owners if they have any difficulties at any point.
- Teach owners how to monitor blood glucose levels at home if required.

The nutritional aims that need to be considered when altering the diet of the animal include:

- Aiding in the reduction of postprandial hyperglycaemic spikes
- Maintaining optimal body condition scores and hydration levels
- Supplying the required amounts of nutrients and calories for the specific life stage, including those lost through clinical symptoms (e.g. the water-soluble vitamins if polyuria is present).

Diabetic nurse clinic protocol

Having a protocol for the diabetic clinic can be useful (see Chapter 6). Having a checklist to run through (see Box 25.2) can help the veterinary nurse to ensure that all points have been covered, and specific notes can be added where greater clarification is required by the owner.

Box 25.2   Diabetic clinic protocol

1 All newly diagnosed diabetic cases should be discharged by the diabetic care nurse, with a 30–45 minute appointment allocated.
2 Subjects to discuss with the owner include: how to give injections, storage of insulin, disposal of sharps and monitoring of the animal. This includes polydipsia and polyuria, appetence levels, lethargy, activity levels, how to identify hypoglycaemic episodes. The treatment of hypoglycaemic episodes and what to do if the owner is worried at any point should be covered. Symptoms of hypoglycaemia should be included, but this does not necessarily mean that all will be noted by the owner:

Polyphagia
Weakness/lethargy
Disorientation
Ataxia

(Continued)

Strange behaviour, e.g. aimless wandering (sometimes noted as being vacant), searching for food, licking lips

Severe neurological signs, e.g., collapse, convulsions, loss of consciousness and eventually death

3   If required, the process of home monitoring can be discussed, and the owner shown how to use a glucometer. A second appointment can be made to cover this subject if the owner wants to have two consultations, as it can be a large amount of information to take on board in one session. Literature or DVDs on this subject can be useful for the client to take away and view before the second nurse consultation.

4   Discuss how the diabetes stabilisation programme works. Explain why the insulin levels are only increased once every 7–10 days in small increments followed by glucose curve until the correct dose is reached. Explain to the owner that it can take a long time, so that they are not disheartened if it does take a while to stabilise.

5   Discuss exercise regimes and feeding levels and timings. It can also be useful to discuss what to do if the animal is unwell, or has not eaten all of its diet. Again, it can be a little overwhelming for owners with newly diagnosed animals to have all of this information. Splitting up the information into two consultations a week apart can be useful.

6   Discuss the type of diet the animal is receiving. If the pet is already receiving a 'good' diet, then it can remain on the diet. If not, especially it is a semi-moist diet, the animal's diet will need to be changed. Semi-moist diets are higher in simple sugars and can cause higher postprandial hyperglycaemic spikes than any other diets. Ideally the pet should transition on to a diet specifically designed for diabetic animals as this can have several benefits.

7   Ensure that the owner has business card/contact details of the diabetes nurse in charge of the case. Having a named nurse can greatly increase compliance, and ease any worries that the owner may have. Ensure that the owners are aware that in an emergency they are not to wait until the diabetic nurse is next on duty, but should phone the practice as soon as possible. The use of email can be just as helpful as a phone number in order to contact the diabetic nurse.

8   Fill out a diabetes care sheet, and explain to the owner how to fill out the diabetes diary. This is very helpful if more than one person is caring for the animal, so that the pet is not accidentally injected more than once. Having written instructions is very important with all new cases.

9   The diabetes nurse in charge of the case should contact the owner for the first couple of days to ensure that the owner is happy with injecting insulin. If not, the owner and pet can come to the practice for the first few injections with the nurse present to help if required.

Clinical nutrition

Water

Polydipsia (excessive drinking) and polyuria (passing excessive amounts of urine) are clinical symptoms of diabetes mellitus. Obligatory losses of electrolytes, such as sodium, potassium, chloride, calcium and phosphorus, and the water-soluble vitamins will occur. Access to fresh water at all times is required, and in severe cases administration of parenteral fluid may be required. Monitoring fluid intake, if possible, is a good indicator of glucose control, and insulin effect. Diabetic diaries are a good idea, and if owners can comment on daily water consumption this can be helpful when stabilising patients.

Proteins

Protein levels may need to be increased for diabetic dogs, especially in the quality of the proteins provided. This is due to loss of amino acids in the urine, a consequence of renal glomerulopathy, or changes in hormonal signals. However, excess protein levels need to be avoided, as renal damage can be enhanced. For diabetic cats the protein and carbohydrate balance is an important factor in clinical nutrition.

Carbohydrates

Consumption of soluble or simple carbohydrates is the primary cause of rapid postprandial hyperglycaemic spikes. Diets need not to include high levels of soluble carbohydrates and the feeding of treats high in soluble carbohydrates should be stopped. The use of insoluble carbohydrates (i.e. fibre) has a positive effect on glycaemic control in dogs and cats. Diets that contain fibre, which exerts gelling properties, can slow the rate of presentation of nutrients (including glucose) to the body. This helps reduce the postprandial spike. The fermentation products of fibre, short-chain or volatile fatty acids, also modify the secretion of some of the digestive hormones and the sensitivity of tissues to insulin. Complex carbohydrates should provide about 50–60% of the calories in diets for dogs, and for cats that are being fed a high-fibre diet (Michel 2005).

Felines are obligate carnivores, and have a unique metabolism. Initially, a growth diet was the diet of choice for diabetic cats, because of the relative increased protein content and decreased carbohydrate content. Now, specific diets for diabetic cats are widely available. For owners who cannot afford a prescription diet, a good-quality kitten diet can still be recommended. A decrease in carbohydrate content will also create a relative increase in the dry matter percentage of fat content (Table 25.1).

A high-protein, low-carbohydrate diet has shown to enhance insulin sensitivity. Blood glucose levels should be monitored after introduction of the diet, as hypoglycaemia can result. This combination of high levels of protein and low levels of carbohydrate closely resembles the natural diet of a cat in the wild. Studies examining this dietary therapy have shown that insulin treatments could be discontinued in 15 out of 24 cats (Mazzaferro et al. 2003).

Vitamins and minerals

Polyuria (a common clinical symptom of diabetes) will increase the loss of electrolytes and water-soluble vitamins, with magnesium and phosphorus being the most significantly lost. Chromium can be used to improve peripheral insulin

Table 25.1   Difference between a traditionally used high-fibre diet compared to a high-protein, low-carbohydrate diet for cats with diabetes

Diet	Carbohydrate		Protein		Fat		Fibre	
	DM(%)	g/100 kcal	DM(%)	g/100 kcal	DM(%)	g/100 kcal	DM(%)	g/100 kcal
Hills w/d	25	6.5	41	11	17	4.4	10.7	2.9
Hills m/d	15.7	3.9	52.8	13	19.4	4.8	6	1.5
Difference	62%↓	60%↓	24%↑	15%↑	13↑	9%↑	56%↓	51%↓

DM, dry matter.

sensitivity and glucose tolerance, though accurate studies on the use of chromium have not been conclusive. Vanadium, when dosed in pharmacological amounts, has insulin-like effects, though it causes gastrointestinal side effects, and chronic excessive intake may have toxic effects.

Feeding a diabetic pet

Dramatic changes to an animal's diet can be indicated when it is diagnosed with diabetes mellitus. A high-carbohydrate diet should be avoided, as should semi-moist diets. These diets have a hyperglycaemic effect because of the increased levels of simple carbohydrates and other ingredients used as humectants (e.g. propylene glycol).

Cost plays a deciding factor in choosing a diet for a diabetic patient, as does whether or not the animal eats the food. High-fibre diets are exceptionally useful in aiding stabilisation of glucose control in dogs, but if the dog is unwilling to consume adequate amounts, this can be detrimental to the animal. An underweight animal will need a modified diet in order to gain weight, but this can only be achieved with insulin therapy.

Administration of exogenous insulin needs to be coordinated with times of feeding. Insulin regimes, whether insulin is being administered once or twice daily, will have a large effect on quantities being fed at each mealtime. If insulin is injected once daily, half the food should be fed at the time of injection, the remainder 8–10 hours later. Twice-daily injections require meals containing half the daily calorific intake at the same time as insulin administration. The owner needs to be aware of the detrimental effects of feeding snacks and treats between meals. Milk should also be avoided because of its calorific content.

The timing of meals is not as critical in feline diabetic patients, and it is advised to continue feeding the cat in the way that it is used to (e.g. *ad libitum*). Cats that are fed set meals should receive one third of the daily food requirement at the time of administration of insulin. The remainder of the diet should be fed at the estimated peak action time of the insulin (when the nadir occurs); this differs for each animal.

In cases of hypoglycaemia the owner can administer dextrose gel (Hypo-stop gel), or honey, jam or syrup, to the mucous membranes of the mouth. This should only be recommended on advice from the veterinary surgeon once the owner has contacted the veterinary practice, or the blood glucose level has been measured. Use of a glucometer at home can be exceptionally useful, but obtaining sufficient blood for a test during a hypoglycaemic episode can be very difficult because of constriction of the peripheral blood supply, and in more severe cases shaking or convulsions. Depending on glycaemic control, smaller frequent meals may prove to be more beneficial in obtaining control. The use of mini-glucose curves in establishing nadir, length of insulin action and dietary effect is invaluable.

Feeding an insulin-resistant obese cat

Many cats that present with type 2 diabetes are obese (Stogdale 1986). A controlled weight loss programme is required in these cases. Predisposition to hepatic lipidosis during rapid weight loss is of concern in cats. Once an ideal BCS has been achieved, and glucose levels remain stable, it is important that these animals receive regular check-ups, including weighing and fructosamine levels. Use of a higher fat and protein and lower carbohydrate diet has proved to be very useful in cats suffering from type 2 diabetes.

The choice of diet will also depend on any secondary medical conditions. Renal dysfunction is commonly experienced when there has been a persistent hyperglycaemia. A low-salt diet would be preferable, but care is needed as these diets have higher carbohydrate content because of their restricted protein levels.

Key points

- Establish the correct BCS and lean body mass.
- When establishing an insulin regime, only ever change one factor (e.g. food, insulin levels, timings, etc.) at a time. These changes must be maintained for at least 1 week before to a second change, as the body's physiological response takes time to fully adapt.
- Ensure plenty of fresh water is available to the animal at all times.

References

Mazzaferro EM, Greco DS, Turner AS, Fettman MJ. Treatment of feline diabetes mellitus using an α-glucosidase inhibitor and a low carbohydrate diet. *J Feline Med Surg* 2003; 5(3).

Michel KE. Nutritional management of endocrine disease. In: Ettinger SJ and Feldman EC, eds. *Textbook of Veterinary Internal Medicine*, volume 1, 6th edition. St Louis, MO: Elsevier Science, 2005.

Stogdale L. Definition of diabetes mellitus. *Cornell Vet* 1986; 76:156–174.

Useful resources

Feline Advisory Bureau. www.fabcats.org.uk

26 Epilepsy

Owning an animal that has been diagnosed with epilepsy can be extremely stressful for owners. Owners can find animals suffering from seizures distressing, and very upsetting. In many cases these cases will only be referred to nursing clinics for routine blood sampling in order to check therapeutic levels of anticonvulsants, and organ function that can be affected by these pharmaceuticals. There are many other aspects that the owner can be supported with.

Nurse clinics

The aims of the nurse clinic are:

- To ensure that the client is able to administer any pharmaceuticals, and that any pharmaceuticals are administered at the correct intervals
- To do any sampling required by the veterinary surgeon
- To give guidance on nutrition, any behavioural changes and weight gain associated with the administration of some anticonvulsants.

Pharmaceuticals

Phenobarbital (a member of the barbiturate family) is the most commonly used pharmaceutical for the control of convulsions in dogs and cats. Some 60–80% of epileptic dogs are successfully controlled on phenobarbital alone; for those that are not controlled adequately, potassium bromide can be included in the medication regime. When monitoring serum phenobarbital levels it is important that the blood sample is taken 4–8 hours after the medication was administered. Blood samples should be collected in plain tubes, rather than serum gel tubes, as gel samples can interfere with the test assays, giving inaccurate results. For all serum samples, the sample should be allowed to clot for a minimum of 15 minutes

The Consulting Veterinary Nurse, First Edition. Nicola Ackerman.
© 2012 John Wiley & Sons, Ltd. Published 2012 by John Wiley & Sons, Ltd.

and the sample then spun. The serum should be drawn off form the sample and placed into a second plain tube.

Phenobarbital has side effects, and these also need to be regularly monitored when performing blood sampling. Biochemistry panels with the liver enzymes gamma-glutamyl transpeptidase (GGT), alanine aminotransferase (ALT) and alkaline phosphatase (ALP) should be done every 3–4 months to monitor liver function because of the side effects associated with this medication. All animals should be pre-starved prior to blood sampling but as hyperlipidaemia is often seen in these cases, the animal may require pre-starving for a longer period of time so that they are not too lipaemic to be tested.

Phenobarbital inhibits seizures by decreasing the activity of neurons. Unfortunately, this effect is not specific to the neurons involved in the seizures but affects other neurons as well. Many of the potential side effects of this drug are caused by this effect on neurons. These side effects can include sedation, lethargy, excessive urination, excessive thirst and excessive hunger, hyperexcitability, ataxia (loss of coordination or hind end weakness) and restlessness. Most of these side effects diminish or disappear after the first few weeks of therapy. Excessive urination, excessive thirst and excessive hunger are the most common long-term side effects.

Clinical nutrition

The clinical nutrition for animals with epilepsy needs to reflect the life stage, and any other potential concurrent medical conditions. Due to the potential side effects of phenobarbital medications, a diet that will help support hepatic function and reduce any potential hyperlidaemia will be of benefit. For details on clinical nutrition regarding hepatic support and low-fat diets reference should be made to the relevant chapters.

FAQs for owners of epileptic animals

What should I do if I miss a dose or am late in administering it?

The dose should be administered as soon as possible. As there are peaks and troughs in the blood serum levels of the anticonvulsants there is a requirement for the anticonvulsant and therefore it will still be required to be given.

What should I do if I will not be able to administer the medication at the required time?

Cat feeders that open at a specific time can be used in these situations. Placing the medication in some highly palatable food will encourage the dog to eat the food and tablet. If this system is to be used, the owner needs to be sure that the dog really does eat the tablet.

Should my epileptic pet be on a protein-restricted diet?

There has been some anecdotal evidence that protein-restricted diets aid in controlling seizures in human epileptic suffers. There has also been evidence that high-protein, high-fat diets can also aid in controlling seizures. As yet, no scientific studies have been conducted on animals concerning dietary protein levels and epilepsy.

Should my epileptic pet be on a salt-restricted diet?

Animals that are receiving potassium bromide as part of their medications can benefit from a lower-salt diet. This is because the dietary salt binds with the potassium bromide, lowering its efficiency. A common occurrence is a previous controlled epileptic dog having seizures after being on the beach. If the dog consumes large amounts of salt water the bromide will become bound to the sea salt and again become ineffective in its role as a medication.

My pet is on medications, and has been recommended a high-fibre diet; won't the fibre content effect the medication?

Some medications can be bound by dietary fibre. In these cases it is advisable to administer the diet at a different time from the medication.

Key points

- Maintain optimal weight, as therapeutics can encourage weight gain.
- Aid in the owner in compliance with administering medications, and the timings of medications.
- Make the owner aware of the importance of frequent monitoring.

27 Gastrointestinal Disorders

Many patients are referred to nurse clinics for nutritional advice regarding gastrointestinal problems. The aims of the nurse clinic will depend on a number of issues, such as whether the problem is acute or chronic problems and what the specific ailment is,

- To conduct diagnostic procedures
- To ensure regular weight and body condition score (BCS) are being conducted and the scores are maintained
- To aid the veterinary surgeon in seeing if any treatments have been successful
- To support the client, answering any questions that they may have.

Diagnostic monitoring

Diagnostic monitoring of these patients is important and can be used to assess efficacy of any treatments, whether pharmaceutical or nutritional. Commonly performed diagnostics would include blood sampling and faecal sampling. More details of different monitoring methods can be found in Chapter 4.

Pharmaceuticals

Many different pharmaceuticals can be used in the treatment of the many different gastrointestinal problems that can be seen in veterinary practice. It is important when conducting nursing clinics to read the clinical history and to make note of the medication regimes that the veterinary surgeon has prescribed for the animal. In some chronic cases drug dosages are tapered to effect and support from the veterinary nurse may be required in order to help clients achieve this.

The Consulting Veterinary Nurse, First Edition. Nicola Ackerman.
© 2012 John Wiley & Sons, Ltd. Published 2012 by John Wiley & Sons, Ltd.

Vitamin B_{12} (cobalamin) injections are commonly used in animals with low blood cobalamin, which is often seen in animals with gastrointestinal problems. In some cases weekly injections may be required for a number of weeks, and this is a role for the veterinary nurse to undertake.

Clinical nutrition

The clinical nutrition for specific gastrointestinal disorders is discussed separately below.

Adverse gastrointestinal reactions to food

Food allergies (food hypersensitivity) have an immunological basis, and cause an adverse reaction to food or a food additive. Food intolerances are abnormal but non-immunological physiological responses to food or a food additive (Buffington et al. 2004). Specific food additives that are known to cause problems include onions and propylene glycol, which can cause haematological abnormalities in cats. Lactose intolerance is a relatively common metabolic adverse reaction in dogs and cats. Diarrhoea can develop when these animals are given cow's or goat's milk, because the lactose content is higher than that of bitch's or queen's milk. Gluten-sensitive enteropathy has been well documented in Irish setters.

The role of food allergies in canine and feline inflammatory bowel disease (IBD) in unknown. It is thought that hypersensitivity to food is involved in the pathogenesis of this syndrome. The role of elimination food trials often alleviate the signs of IBD, which seems to imply that food allergies or food intolerances play a role in this syndrome (Buffington et al. 2004).

For further information on clinical nutrition for patients suffering from adverse food reactions, see Chapter 32.

Acute gastroenteritis and vomiting, or small bowel diarrhoea

Acute vomiting and diarrhoea is the most common reason why animals are presented to the veterinary practice. The definition of diarrhoea is an abnormal increase in frequency, water content or volume of faeces. This can result in the reduced absorption of nutrients, and the loss of water, electrolytes and water-soluble nutrients, which can lead to dehydration and acidosis. Acute diarrhoea can be subdivided into four different categories, as described in detail in Table 27.1.

Acute diarrhoea and vomiting is most commonly due to irritation of the gut mucosa by toxins and infections. The clinical symptoms of vomiting and diarrhoea are a response to remove the causal agent from the gastrointestinal (GI) tract. In some cases abrupt changes to the animal's diet can induce these symptoms. In these cases it is wise to stop feeding the new diet; once the animal has returned to full

Table 27.1 Classification and pathophysiology of diarrhoea

Classification of acute diarrhoea	Pathophysiology	Common causes
Osmotic	Excess water-soluble molecules in the intestinal lumen result in osmotic retention of water. D+ occurs when the fluid volume overwhelms the absorptive capacity of the small intestine and colon	Sudden dietary change, malabsorption
Permeability (exudative)	Inflammation in the intestine can stimulate increase secretion of fluid and electrolytes, and impair absorption	Permeability can be affected by ulceration, especially in cases of neoplastic disease. Where severe damage is present serum protein and blood loss can also occur. Portal hypertension can also result in exudation of fluid into the intestinal lumen
Secretory	When the absorptive capacities of the small intestine and colon are exceeded. Resulting D+ can be severe, and does not usually resolve with fasting	Toxin release by enteric infectious agents (e.g. *Giardia* spp., *Escherichia coli*)
Dysmotility	D+ can result in secondary alterations in motility, usually reduced intestinal motility	Ileus and abnormal dilation of the intestine can be physical, neuromuscular, metabolic or functional abnormalities, and can further promote D+ as stasis allows for bacterial fermentation

D+, diarrhoea.
Source: Battersby and Harvey (2006).

health on the old diet, a slow and correct transitional change can be initiated. It is important to differentiate between small and large intestinal diarrhoea, as treatment can vary (Table 27.2).

Dietary management of cases of acute gastroenteritis, when vomiting is present, can initially include a period of starvation for 24–48 hours; this food deprivation allows the gastrointestinal tract to clear itself of the luminal contents, including the causal agents. It also aids in preventing mucosal cell abrasion, deprives opportunistic pathogenic bacterial of nutrients, preventing absorption of dietary antigens by a compromised mucosa, and may permit re-establishment of brush border enzymatic function.

When starting to feed the animal again, a highly digestible diet should be given in small, frequent meals. This can be a homemade diet of lean chicken or cottage cheese and rice. Specific veterinary diets offer a more balanced nutritional meal, as they will cater for losses of electrolytes and vitamins lost through vomiting and diarrhoea. Electrolyte imbalances can quickly develop in animals with severe diar-

Table 27.2 Differences between small and large intestinal diarrhoea in the cat and dog

Clinical symptom	Small intestinal diarrhoea	Large intestinal diarrhoea
Blood in faeces	Melena	Haematochezia
Frequency of defecation	Mild increase (<3 × day)	Markedly increased (>3 × day)
Faecal volume	Large quantities	Small quantities
Faecal quality	Loose, watery, 'cow-pie'	Loose to semi-formed, 'jelly-like'
Urgency	Usually absent	Often present
Tenesmus	Rare	Common
Faecal mucus	Rare	Common
Dyschezia	Absent	May be present
Vomiting	May be present	May be present
Weight loss	Common	Rare
Flatus/borborygmi	May be present	May be present

Table 27.3 Typical analysis of baby rice

Nutrient	g/100 g (as fed)
Fat	0.8
Fibre	1.5
Carbohydrates (as sugars)	85.6
Protein	8
Water	4

rhoea. Intravenous supplementation should also be provided when required, especially if the animal is vomiting (Battersby and Harvey 2006). Baby rice is an ideal carbohydrate source to use in these cases (Table 27.3), but cats are less tolerant of carbohydrates and more tolerant of fats. An appropriate diet for them would be boiled chicken, or a specific veterinary diet.

Adsorbents are frequently used in these cases, and can be provided with the addition of pro- and prebiotics, and glutamine. The purpose of adsorbents is to bind bacteria and toxins, to protect the intestinal mucosa, and potentially for an antisecretory effect (Battersby and Harvey 2006). Kaolin has been traditionally used, but montmorillonite has been reported to be 20 times more effective than kaolin at adsorbing pathogens (Battersby and Harvey 2006).

Feeding through

In human medicine there is a continuing bank of evidence indicating that 'feeding through' diarrhoea with an appropriate diet can be beneficial. Comparisons can be difficult, as many cases of diarrhoea in humans tend to be secretory, whereas osmotic diarrhoea is more common in dogs and cats (McCann and Simpson 2006). The advantages of feeding through include maintaining mucosal health, reducing the risk of bacterial translocation and aiding in the 'flushing out' of the causal factor. Feeding through should not be used in animals that are vomiting or severely dehydrated. With animals that are vomiting, or if the gastrointestinal tract is not functioning, the animal's nutritional requirements should be met through parenteral nutrition. The obvious disadvantage is the risk of 'accidents' in the house, and the increase in faecal volume. Whether food is withheld or not, unlimited access to water must be maintained at all times. The use of oral rehydration solutions containing carbohydrates, peptides and electrolytes should be advocated in these cases. When using this method, feeding a diet that will not cause an inflammatory reaction in the future is important. Dietary antigens can cross the compromised gastrointestinal mucosa and set up a hypersensitivity reaction. Use of a novel protein and/or carbohydrate source should be recommended. Once the animal is then well, and transferred back to its original diet, it is unlikely to have any reactions to the original protein source.

Anal glands and impactions

Anal gland impactions can occur when the dog's or cat's diet is low or restricted in fibre. The inclusion of fibre in the diet aids as a bulking agent, and allows a constant pressure on the glands at defecation, thus decreasing the risk of the glands becoming full. Glands that become overfull have a higher risk of becoming infected and/or impacted. Dietary management of these cases is necessary, and the inclusion of fibre into the diet is warranted. This can be achieved by feeding a diet higher in fibre, or by the addition of fibre-containing pellets.

Where anal gland surgery has been performed the temporary use of a low-residue (low-fibre) diet is advocated, in order to remove pressure from suture lines.

Borborygmus and flatulence

Borborygmus and flatulence is a very common occurrence in many dogs. This can be due to the diet itself, or the rapid consumption of the diet, which leads to aerophagia. Diets that are low in quality and poorly digestible can be problematic, and dietary change can be recommended in these cases. For dogs that eat their food too quickly, the diet can be spread out on a flat surface, or fed little and often. Adding water to the diet can also aid in increasing consumption time.

Dietary management is concerned with decreasing the production of intestinal gas caused by bacterial fermentation of undigested foods. Diets high in protein may contribute to increased levels of flatulence, as may vitamin and mineral supplements, due to the increased intestinal microbial activity they cause (Davenport et al. 2000). Commercial products are available for reducing flatulence. These products may contain alpha-galactosidase, and reduce flatulence by improving digestion of non-absorbable carbohydrates (Davenport et al. 2000). Other veterinary medicines can contain antacids, aluminium hydroxide and magnesium trisilicate as well as copper complexes of chlorophyllins. Clinical trials have clearly demonstrated the efficacy of these medications in reducing wind and smells and relieving indigestion and gastric upset in the dog. The local antacid effect in the stomach promotes coalescence and removal of trapped gases from the gut contents, thereby limiting their passage through to the later stages of the gastrointestinal tract.

Chronic diarrhoea

Chronic diarrhoea can be a clinical symptom of a vast number of different problems. It is essential to determine the underlying cause so that specific treatments for each individual case can be initiated. Dietary management plays an important role in long-term management of these cases, as relapses can be frequent. As each case is different there is no one specific diet aimed at animals suffering from chronic diarrhoea. Low-fat, single (novel) protein diets may be recommended, but in some cases a diet with a high fibre content is the diet of choice in resolving the clinical symptoms. Chronic diarrhoea disorders such as IBD, protein-losing enteropathy (PLE), antibiotic-responsive diarrhoea (ARD) and irritable bowel syndrome (IBS) are discussed separately because of their significance in veterinary medicine.

Inflammatory bowel disease

The management of IBD involves the combined use of anti-inflammatory medication alongside the use of a single novel protein diet. A full dietary history (see Appendix 1) is required in order to ascertain what protein sources the animal has been exposed to in the past. Diets that contain novel protein sources such as venison or duck have proved to be beneficial. Initially lamb was used as a novel protein source, but many life stage diets now include lamb and are marketed for animals with sensitive stomachs. When using an elimination diet it is important to challenge the system to see if the original diet was the initial cause. See 'Feeding an elimination diet' in Chapter 32 for further details.

The use of fermentable fibre in these cases should not be underestimated. Colonic bacteria easily digest fermentable fibres, which in turn produce butyrate, a short-chain fatty acid (SCFA). Butyrate is the primary energy source for colonic bacteria, and thus helps to maintain gut health. Other SCFAs are also produced, which reduce the colonic pH, and thus reduce the risk of pathogenic bacteria colonising the area. As the body absorbs the SCFA there is an increase in the absorption of electrolytes and water from the colon.

When feeding an animal with IBD the nutritional goal is to provide adequate nutrient intake in order to meet the requirements of the individual, but also to compensate for ongoing losses through the gastrointestinal tract.

Protein-losing enteropathy and lymphangiectasia

Lymphangiectasia is characterised by abnormalities of the intestinal lymphatic system. The condition can be as a primary defect of the lymphatic system, or secondary as a consequence of severe intestinal infiltrative disease (e.g. IBD, lymphosarcoma; Elwood 1998). Lymphangiectasia is the most common cause of PLE in dogs and cats. Not all animals present with the clinical symptom of diarrhoea, but they often present with progressive weight loss even with a good calorific consumption. The leaky intestinal lymphatics result in hypoalbuminaemia and loss of colloidal oncotic pressure.

When feeding animals with PLE the key is to control dietary fat levels. Long-chain triglycerides provide a major stimulus for intestinal lymph flow; the protein content of the lymph tends to increase with the dietary fat content. Limiting dietary fat content will reduce the lymphatic flow, reduces lacteal and lymphatic distension and thus minimise protein losses (Elwood 1998). Dietary fat levels of less than 10% DMB for dogs and less than 15% DMB for cats is recommended (Elwood 1998). The protein level of the diet is important; feeding a high-protein diet has been shown to be unsuccessful. The cause of the PLE is important, as in cases where severe IBD is the underlying cause; care should be given when selecting a protein source. Dietary protein should be of a high biological value, and levels in excess of 25% DMB for dogs and in excess of 35% DMB in cats have been recommended (Elwood 1998).

Antibiotic-responsive diarrhoea

ARD should be best managed with a combination of antibiotics and diet. The response to antibiotics will dictate the length of the course required. The antibiotics of choice in cases of ARD are tylosin or oxytetracycline (King 2005). Little research has been conducted on the casual factors of ARD, but it is speculated that gastrointestinal factors must promote bacterial colonies that are causal agents for the diarrhoea. The use of prebiotics has been recommended in these cases in order to promote gastrointestinal health. Dietary manipulation should be considered if the animal is on an inappropriate diet that encourages growth of pathogenic bacteria.

Irritable bowel syndrome

IBS is a difficult disorder to diagnose; only on exclusion of all other causes of chronic diarrhoea can a diagnosis of IBS be made. Clinical signs of IBS include bouts of abdominal pain and chronic large intestinal diarrhoea. The clinical signs can be intermittent, with stress also being a probably trigger factor. The addition of fibre to the diet has proved to be of slight benefit in some cases (Ragni 2005).

Colitis

Colitis (inflammation of the colon) is the most common causes of diarrhoea in dogs and cats. Colitis is characterised by the presence of mucus covering the faeces, and/or fresh blood. There are many causes of colitis, including stress. Many dogs have colitis diarrhoea when being hospitalised at veterinary practices, due to stress levels. Dietary management of mild cases is recommended, though in chronic or severe cases medical treatment may be required alongside dietary management. Modifications to the diet include:

- High-fibre diets that normalise the transit time and bind faecal water (fibre also acts as a prebiotic, aiding the strains and populations of gut bacteria)
- Low-fibre, highly digestible diets which aid in reducing the quantity of undigested food entering the colon
- Hypoallergenic diets, which can also be used when an intolerance or hypersensitivity is present.

When the initiating cause of the colitis is unknown, dietary modifications can be very much a case of trial and error, as the first two options (high-fibre and low-fibre) contradict each other. This should be relayed to owners so that they have a better understanding of the problem, and do not get frustrated with dietary management. It is also recommended to advise owners that colitis is normally seen spasmodically, with intervals of normality between bouts.

Constipation/megacolon

Constipation in animals can be a clinical symptom of systemic disease, a response to nutrition or nutritional changes, or a consequence to damage to the pelvis. Constipation is characterised by absent, infrequent, or difficult defecation associated with retention of faeces within the colon and rectum (Davenport et al. 2000). The treatment and preventive management of constipation varies. The addition of fibre to the diet while the animal is constipated can compound the initial problem. Treatments can include enemas and laxatives. In order to prevent the recurrence of constipation, a full history is required in order to identify the casual factor or factors. The water and fibre consumption of the animal need to be ascertained. Maintenance of normal hydration levels is required; intake of water should be 40–60 mL/kg body weight per day. Recommendations for increasing water intake in animals are detailed in Chapter 12. Fibre intake can be estimated from details on the pet food label.

Increasing the fibre content of the diet can improve constipation dramatically, by increasing the water content of the faeces, intestinal transition rates and colonic motility. When increasing the dietary fibre content of the diet, it should be remembered that both fermentable and non-fermentable fibres should be included. High-fibre foods can be less palatable, and the transition to a fibre-enhanced veterinary therapeutic diet can be difficult. In some cases staying on the original diet but adding a source of fibre can be helpful. Some animals can suffer side effects when changed to a high-fibre diet, if the transition is done too quickly. Flatulence and abdominal cramping are common side effects of the addition of fermentable fibres. Some animals can develop megacolon or constipation when fed a moderate to high fibre diet (>15% DM crude fibre). The transition to these diets should be made by increasing fibre content in gradual increments. If side effects occur, then it is recommended that the fibre content be decreased by 5% DMB and the animal reassessed. Up to 10% fibre can be added to the diet without compromising its overall nutrient balance. Titration of the dietary fibre content of the diet can be achieved by the use of food combinations with diets of varying crude fibre content.

In situations of severe constipation or megacolon where colonic motility is not present, the use of a high-fibre diet is not recommended. In these cases a highly digestible diet (DM digestibility >90%) is the diet of choice. This will have an exceptionally low residue, while still providing adequate calories. In these cases faecal production is sufficiently reduced that removal of the faeces can be achieved via enemas once or twice weekly.

The use of medical therapies in the aid of constipation is important as an adjunct to dietary management, and suitable for mild to moderate constipation. Laxatives such as lactulose, sorbitol and polyethylene glycol are poorly absorbed carbohydrates and prove to be very useful. These sugars are hydrolysed to fatty acids by the colonic microflora, where they exert osmotic pressure and draw fluid into the colonic lumen. Colonic motility modifiers such as cisapride are also useful, especially in rabbits. The dose rate for dogs and cats is 0.25 mg/kg body weight, three or four times a day (Buffington et al. 2004). Treatment of constipation and megacolon in animals is very much case specific, and can be dependent on the initiating case.

Gastric dilation–volvulus

Gastric dilation–volvulus (GDV), or bloat, is thought to be the final common pathway of a variety of problems in certain predisposed large breeds of dogs (Buffington et al. 2004). Gastric dilation is defined as the distension of the stomach with a mixture of air, food and fluid. GDV occurs when the stomach rotates on its mesenteric axis. This entraps the gastric contents, while also compromising the vascular supply to the stomach, spleen and pancreas. Breeds that are predisposed are large breed, deep-chested dogs, including Irish setters, Great Danes, standard poodles, Dobermann pinschers, German shepherds and St Bernards. Dogs with a BCS of 2/5 or less are also considered a risk factor for GDV. Males are twice as likely as females to develop GDV, and having a relative, especially a parent, that has experienced GDV greatly increases the risk, which can be as much as 63% greater if a first-degree relative has suffered from GDV (Ragni 2005). Other dogs that seem to be predisposed to GDV are those which tend to be nervous and stressful. These dogs should always be fed alone, and in a quiet environment.

Diet can play some role in susceptible animals, but no diet-related cause has been clearly identified (Buffington et al. 2004). Several dietary risk factors have been identified, however, and these include:

- Feeding only one meal per day.
- Postprandial exercise, especially vigorous exercise. Recommendations include avoiding exercise 1 hour before a meal and 2 hours after. Gentle exercise has been shown to improve gastrointestinal functioning, but must be restricted.
- Rapid consumption of food, leading to aerophagia. This can be aided by placing the food on a flat baking tray, or spreading the dry food out on the floor.
- Food particle/kibble diameter of less than 30 mm.
- Consumption of large volumes of water. The availability of water immediately after feeding needs to be limited, if consumption is large (more than one volume of water per volume of dry food). Mixing water with the dry diet in equal proportions can help to prevent the consumption of large volumes of water.
- Episodes of overeating.
- All dietary transitions should be done slowly; see Chapter 11 for details.

The consumption of dry diets has been blamed in the past for being a predisposing factor for GDV, but epidemiological studies have shown this to be incorrect (Elwood 1998).

Feeding a dog predisposed to GDV

As no specific nutritional factors have been established for GD or GDV, it is difficult to advise on a specific dietary regime for these animals. The diet needs to provide all the adequate nutrients and energy requirements for the animal's particular life stage. The use of a highly digestible lower-fat diet has been advocated in these situations, as it is less fermentable and will have a shorter transit time through the stomach.

The daily management of the dog is important. This includes dividing the diet into small frequent meals, feeding from a raised level, avoiding exercise around the times of feeding, decreasing competitive feeding, feeding a mixture of moist and dry diets, increasing the time it takes for the dog to consume the diet and avoiding excess water consumption after eating.

Owners should always be advised of the symptoms of GD or GDV in all breeds that are predisposed. In veterinary practices it is advisable to inform clients of this when they initially present their puppies at puppy clinics or for their initial vaccinations.

Hairballs in cats and rabbits

Hairballs are a common occurrence in cats. Animals with longer, thicker coats or those with fastidious grooming behaviour tend to suffer more. Most hairballs do not usually cause clinical disease, though vomiting can be a nuisance or even distressing for owners. Laxatives and lubricants can be utilised, either with or without specialised diets, for the routine management of hairballs. The use of lubricants and laxatives should be limited, because they interfere with normal digestion and absorption of nutrients.

Hairballs are loose accumulations of hair and mucus, which form in the digestive tract. In some cases the hair and mucus can coalesce with other materials to form trichobezoars, which are much harder. Trichobezoars form within the stomach or intestines, and are less common in cats but are a common cause of anorexia in rabbits. If the trichobezoars become large enough, obstruction of the pyloric or intestines can occur. Hairballs are a common finding in rabbits because of their inability to vomit, and should be considered even in short-haired animals which present with anorexia. Often a large doughy mass can be felt on palpation of the stomach. Treatment for trichobezoars is based on breaking down the proteinaceous matrix that binds them together. Large trichobezoars must be removed via surgery or endoscopy (Buffington et al. 2004). If they are left, obstructions and ileus can occur (Krempels et al. 2000). Survival after surgery of the digestive tract, particularly gastrotomy, is reportedly low in rabbits (Brewer and Cruise 1994). Hairballs in rabbits can be prevented by feeding a diet with adequate dietary fibre (>14% DM crude fibre), minimising stress and boredom, and grooming the animal frequently (Ragni 2005).

A common treatment for hairballs is pineapple juice and papaya juice, the supposed active ingredient being the enzymes bromelin (in pineapple juice) or papain (in papaya juice). There is no evidence to support this, and in truth bromelin and papain are incapable of dissolving keratin, the main protein component of hair (Brewer and Cruise 1994, Watson 2005). Simple sugars in the fruit juices may actually promote overgrowth of *Clostridium* spp. (Watson 2005).

Key points

- Help the client to understand the disease or medical process that the animal may be experiencing.
- Maintain optimal weight and BCS.
- Give appropriate dietary advice, which may include the requirement for diet trials and exclusion diets.

References

Battersby I, Harvey A. Differential diagnosis and treatment of acute diarrhoea in the dog and cat. *In Practice* 2006; 28:480–488.

Brewer NR, Cruise LJ. Physiology. In: Manning PJ, Ringer DH and Newcomer CE, eds. *The Biology of the Laboratory Rabbit*. San Diego, CA: Academic Press, 1994, p. 65.

Buffington T, Holloway C, Abood S. *Manual of Veterinary Dietetics*. St Louis, MO: Elsevier Saunders, 2004.

Davenport DJ, Remillard RL, Simpson KW, Pidgeon GL. Gastrointestinal and exocrine pancreatic disease. In: Hand MS, Thatcher CD, Remillard RL, Roudebush P, eds. *Small*

Animal Clinical Nutrition, 4th edition. Topeka, KS: Mark Morris Institute, 2000, pp. 725–810.

Elwood CM. Risk factors for gastric dilation in Irish setter dogs. *J Small Anim Pract* 1998; 39:185–190.

King C. Gastrointestinal tract and stasis in the rabbit. *VN Times* 2005; Nov:19.

Krempels D, Cotter M, Stanzione G. Ileus in domestic rabbits. *Exotic DVM* 2000; 2.4:19–21.

McCann T, Simpson JW. Approach to the management of diarrhoea. *UK Vet* 2006; 11(6):30–37.

Ragni RA. GDV: Preventing the nightmare is best. *Vet Times* 2005; 31 Oct:6–7.

Watson PJ. Managing canine pancreatitis. *BSAVA Congress Scientific Proceedings*, 2005, pp. 97–99.

28 Hepatobiliary Disorders

The role of the liver in the body is critical in maintaining homeostasis and the removal of waste products that have accumulated within the body. The liver is essential in the production of proteins and deamination of excessive unrequired proteins. Understanding the functioning of the liver is essential in designing a diet relating to the clinical symptoms that the animal is exhibiting. The liver can be damaged in a number of different ways, from infection and hepatic encephalopathy as an adjunct to medical therapies and from toxins (see box). Congenital abnormalities such as portal systemic shunts will also affect the way in which the liver functions. Analysis of laboratory results and other diagnostic means will enable the practitioner to identify where the damage is occurring within the liver. Delayed recovery from general anaesthesia may be the first indication of compromised liver function (see Box 28.1).

Box 28.1   Causes of liver damage

- **Infectious:** leptospirosis, ascending biliary infections, septicaemia
- **Inflammatory:** immune mediated, idiopathic
- **Metabolic (lipidosis):** idiopathic, secondary to starvation
- **Toxic:** drugs, mushroom consumption
- **Idiopathic:** chronic active hepatitis

Nurse clinic

For these patients the nursing clinic is a starting point to discuss nutrition and hepatic supplements. The nutritional management of hepatobiliary disease is usually directed at clinical manifestations of the disease rather than the specific cause itself.

The aims of nutritional management are:

- Maintaining the normal metabolic processes
- Avoiding toxic by-product accumulation
- Correcting any electrolyte disturbances
- Providing substrates that support hepatocellular regeneration and repair.

The Consulting Veterinary Nurse, First Edition. Nicola Ackerman.
© 2012 John Wiley & Sons, Ltd. Published 2012 by John Wiley & Sons, Ltd.

The aims of the nurse clinic are to:

- Discuss the above nutritional recommendations
- Discuss the use of supplements that aid hepatic function
- Monitor body weight and body condition score (BCS)
- Do any diagnostic blood sampling required by the veterinary surgeon.

There is no one 'ideal' liver disease treatment or diet. The dietary needs of the patient require a good understanding of what you are trying to achieve and the individual animal's needs. A palatable, high-quality, protein diet, supplemented with zinc, B vitamins and antioxidants should be fed. Protein should be reduced but not restricted unless it is essential to control encephalopathy. Malnutrition is a very common feature of chronic hepatic disease, and correct nutrition for each individual patient is important to help regulate the hormonal milieu that occurs with hepatic injury.

Clinical nutrition

Protein

The maintenance of a positive nitrogen balance is important for the preservation of body condition and protein synthesis. Protein malnutrition is common in patients with chronic liver disease, where the clinical manifestations include weight loss, loss of muscle tissue and hypoalbuminaemia. Protein intake needs to be finely balanced; in some dogs the protein requirements may exceed those of normal maintenance requirements due to the increased protein turnover and the demands of hepatocellular regeneration. A moderate restriction of protein levels is not always recommended, and the quality (biological value) of the proteins should be increased. This is recommended, as they fulfil the animal's needs with minimal production of nitrogenous waste. Studies in human patients with hepatic failure have shown that the nitrogen balance can be improved if the diet is divided into small, frequent meals.

Dairy products (cottage cheese, milk) or eggs are highly beneficial, probably owing to factors such as the relatively high ratio of carbohydrates to protein and their influence on intestinal transit and colonic pH, as well as the differing amino acid composition. Fibre of soya origin has shown to provide an excellent source of dietary fibre that reduces ammonia production and absorption in the colon and assists ammonia elimination in the faeces.

One of the roles of the liver is protein regulation, including degradation of the essential amino acids, including the aromatic amino acids (AAA) but not the branched-chain amino acids (BCAA), and some of the non-essential amino acids. Dogs and other omnivores are able to down-regulate protein degradation activities when minimal dietary protein is consumed, but cats are not able to do this. Plasma amino acid concentrations differ, depending on the type of hepatic failure. In the normal healthy animal AAA (tyrosine, phenylalanine and tryptophan) are effectively extracted from the portal circulation and metabolised by the liver. Reduced hepatic function is associated with an increase in circulating AAA. Conversely the plasma concentrations of BCAA (leucine, isoleucine and valine) and most other amino acids are reduced due to an increased rate of metabolising by muscle and adipose tissue. The ratio between AAA and BCAA can be used in order to evaluate the liver function. In healthy dogs the ratio between BCAA and AAA ranges between 3.0 and 4.0, but the ratio can be reduced to 1.0 or less in dogs with portosystemic vascular anomalies and chronic hepatitis. Other factors such as increased levels of insulin, glucagons and catecholamines are thought to contribute to the altered amino acid metabolism seen in these patients. Alterations in this ratio have also been implicated in the pathogenesis of hepatic encephalopathy. Hence BCAA-enriched solutions have been used in human nutritional support for many years in those patients suffering from chronic hepatic disease and hepatic encephalopathy.

Carbohydrates and fats

Non-protein calories should come from highly digestible carbohydrate and fat sources. The fat level in the diet should not be restricted unless there is clinical evidence of steatorrhoea.

Vitamins and minerals

The requirement of vitamins and minerals within the diet is dependent on the causal problem with the liver. Copper levels should be restricted due to accumulation within the liver, and is discussed further below. Vitamins, which are produced within the liver, should be supplemented, as deficiencies are common, as is a deficiency of zinc. Due to the oxidative cell damage, which is correlated with the severity of liver disease, antioxidants should also be supplemented.

Copper-associated hepatotoxicosis in dogs

Bedlington terriers can often develop copper storage disease and subsequently hepatitis and cirrhosis. Statistics indicate that roughly 25% of Bedlington terriers are affected and another 50% are carriers. Some other breeds that have also been affected are West Highland white terriers and Dobermann pinschers. Copper-associated hepatotoxicosis is caused by an inherited autosomal recessive trait that results in impaired biliary excretion of copper. Diets for these dogs need to have reduced levels of copper, and supplements containing copper should also be avoided. Homemade diets should not contain liver, shellfish or organ meats, which are all high in copper content.

The role of copper in hepatic diseases in other breeds of dogs is less clear. There are theories that elevated hepatic copper concentrations precede liver damage, whereas others contend that the excess hepatic copper results from faulty copper excretion caused by chronic cholestasis. A third theory is that elevated levels are antecedent to the disease and are incidental to disease progression. Anti-inflammatory agents, such as prednisolone, can be beneficial in the management of chronic hepatitis in Bedlington terriers and West Highland white terriers.

The nutritional aims of managing patients with copper-associated hepatotoxicosis are:

- To further decrease absorption of copper from the gastrointestinal tract
- To enhance copper excretion.

Portal systemic shunts and hepatic encephalopathy

Portal systemic shunts (PSS) are vascular communications between the portal and systemic venous systems. This communication allows access of portal blood to the systemic circulation without passing through the liver. Congenital PSS are most common and are inherited. They may either be intrahepatic (in large breeds such as Irish wolfhound and Burmese mountain dog) or extrahepatic (in medium and toy breeds, such as Yorkshire terrier, cairn terrier and dachshund). Stunted growth or failure to gain weight can occur in these animals. Acquired PSS forms in response to portal hypertension caused by fibrosis and chronic cirrhosis. As a result of inadequate hepatic clearance of toxins and altered liver function, hepatic encephalopathy can result. Ammonium urate and other purine uroliths can also occur due to the high urinary excretion of ammonia and uric acid.

Shunting results in nutritional depletion of the liver as well as failed delivery of substrates to the liver for degradation and metabolism. Hepatic encephalopathy (HE) is a complex metabolic disorder, which is characterised by abnormal mental status. There are many factors that can precipitate HE (see Box 28.2).

Box 28.2 Factors precipitating hepatic encephalopathy (HE)

- High-protein meal
- Gastrointestinal bleeding or ingestion of blood
- Transfusion of stored blood
- Constipation
- Azotaemia
- Metabolic alkalosis
- Hypokalaemia
- Dietary methionine
- Catabolism/hypermetabolism
- Sedatives/anaesthetics

The nutritional aims for managing patients with HE include:

- Reducing dietary protein
- Changing intestinal flora
- Decreasing intestinal transit time.

Soluble or fermentable fibre in the diet such as cellulose and lactulose will aid the animal's suffering from liver dysfunction as it helps reduce the side effects of deamination of proteins. Lactulose is a synthetic disaccharide that is metabolised into volatile short-chain fatty acids in the colon. The change in the lumen pH traps the ammonia as ammonium ions, which are removed in the faeces. There is also the beneficial effect that colonic bacteria use the increased nitrogen in reproduction and growth, while also inhibiting ammonia generation by colonic bacteria through a process known as catabolite repression.

Insoluble or non-fermentable fibre is also an important constituent in the diet of animals suffering from hepatic disease. Constipation is a predisposing factor for the development of encephalopathy since it increases the contract time for colonic bacteria to act on the faeces and produce ammonia.

Vitamins and minerals

Vitamin E is a superb antioxidant, and may be cytoprotective especially in copper toxicity; due to the effects it has protecting against lipid peroxidation. Vitamin K supplementation may become a necessity if clotting times are prolonged, especially prior to hepatic biopsies being taken. The vitamin K stores within the liver are eliminated and do become rapidly depleted, although the function for synthesis of the prothrombin-complex clotting factors is always lost before the storage of vitamin K is depleted. The other fat-soluble vitamins of A and D should not be supplemented, as vitamin A can cause hepatic damage and vitamin D can cause calcification within the tissues.

The level of calorific intake determines the requirements for the water-soluble vitamins. Thus if anorexia is present the requirement is low, though when nutrition intake increases, the water-soluble vitamins are required in order to replenish coenzymes involved in metabolic processes in the liver and other tissues. As with all animals suffering from polydipsia and polyuria, supplementation with B vitamins is required. Animals suffering from hepatic disease have been recommended to receive a double dose of B vitamins. Vitamin C should not be supplemented as it can increase the tissue damage associated with copper and iron disease.

Choline is essential in the packaging of VLDL (very low-density lipoproteins) in the liver and therefore the exportation of triglycerides. A choline deficiency with concurrent lipolysis may slow down VLDL export and promote hepatic lipid accumulation. Hepatic diets should contain supplementation of choline and carnitine, but the efficacy levels are unknown.

There are large amounts of supportive data indicating that zinc deficiency is common with hepatic injury. This is due to a reduction in absorption and an increase loss via the urine. Nutrition supplementation of the diet with zinc reduces encephalopathy; at an effective rate the same as lactulose.

Feeding a hepatic diet

The aim of the dietary modifications is to meet the animal's daily requirement for nutrients, whilst reducing the metabolic demands placed upon the liver. The calorific needs of the liver should be met with non-protein calories and the nutritional deficiencies which can occur due to the loss of hepatic function, need to be met within the diet

Frequent feeding of small meals is preferred to ensure optimal assimilation and to limit the entry of dietary protein into the colon. Other complications of liver disease include gastrointestinal ulceration and ascites. If ulceration is known to be present the animal must not go without food.

Idiopathic feline hepatic lipidosis

The incidence rate of feline hepatic lipidosis is unfortunately increasing. Most of these cats are obese and usually present with a history of prolonged anorexia after a stressful event. Hepatic lipidosis is characterised by accumulation of excess triglycerides in the hepatocytes, which results in cholestasis and hepatic dysfunction. This disease may be idiopathic or may develop secondary to some underlying medical problem. Hepatic lipidosis is more commonly seen in cats because there are several features of cat metabolism that make them less tolerant to periods of anorexia. For example, the cat's ability to synthesise the amino acid arginine is lower than that of other species. This amino acid is an intermediate of the urea cycle, in which ammonia is converted to urea. Its other role is in the production of apoproteins, which are incorporated in VLDL. VLDL transport triglycerides from the liver to adipose tissue. Any changes in the availability of arginine can result in hyperammonaemia, even when there is minimal hepatic dysfunction, and disturbance to the transport of triglycerides. Taurine is also required in VLDL production and the conjunction of bile acids. As taurine is also required in larger amounts in the cat, any deficiencies can result in VLDL disturbances. L-Carnitine is also essential in the transportation of long-chained fatty acids into the mitochondria. L-Carnitine is often supplemented into hepatic diets and obesity diets for this reason, aiding in the mobilisation of circulating fats. If any of these supply chains become unbalanced then hepatic lipidosis can occur. Since any disruption in hepatic lipid metabolism can cause lipidosis, it is unlikely that there is a common cause for all cases of feline hepatic lipidosis. Hypokalaemia is present in about 30% of cats with severe hepatic lipidosis, hence electrolyte monitoring is important, as hypokalaemia can prolong anorexia and exacerbate expression of HE.

Insulin resistance with subsequent glucose intolerance represents a key metabolic abnormality in all patients with chronic hepatic injury. This can be due to reduced insulin activity from depletion of insulin receptors on the target cells. This is why many cats with hepatic lipidosis are hyperglycaemic. Reduced insulin activity results in activation of triacylglycerol lipase, with consequent hydrolysis of triglycerols, resulting in the increased release of free fatty acids into the circulation from the adipose tissue.

Treatment of feline hepatic lipidosis

Nutrition plays a supportive role in the management of most hepatic diseases, but for feline idiopathic hepatic lipidosis nutritional therapy is the primary treatment. It is a condition that requires vigorous supportive care, including intravenous fluids and nutritional support. The provision of an adequate daily energy intake is the cornerstone of successful medical management. This is can only truly be achieved through early tube feeding via a nasogastric tube. Force-feeding of the cat or the use of appetite stimulants can work to a degree, but rarely meet the animal's calorific needs.

Food aversion is an exceptionally important component to be considered when tempting anorexic cats, which is why tube feeding is a more preferable method. Intravenous feeding (total parenteral feeding) is not recommended unless some enteral nutrition is also being concurrently provided. Parenteral feeding is associated with hepatic steatosis, villus atrophy, fluid and electrolyte imbalances, and an increased incidence of sepsis. This is due to enteral nutrition providing antigenic stimulation to the gut-associated lymphoid tissue (GALT) and stimulating secretion of IgA, which helps to maintain an intact gastrointestinal barrier, in order to prevent bacterial translocation. Other factors that need to be considered in these cases include:

- Correction of hypokalaemia: This can be achieved by potassium supplementation through intravenous fluids and oral, tube feeding methods.
- Correction of hyperglycaemia, and cell intake of calories: Carbohydrates should not replace the dietary fat due to this glucose intolerance.
- Dietary protein intake: This needs to be adapted to suit the individual patient. It is advised that the protein intake should not be reduced below 20% of calories from this source.
- When starting tube feeding a balanced formulation sufficient to meet the cat's resting energy requirement (RER) at its current weight is ideal. Grossly obese cats carrying 35% or more fat should be fed at a lower estimated optimal weight rather than their current weight.

Supplements

Nutraceuticals can be beneficial in a number of hepatic conditions; these include toxicities (pharmaceutical/plant), chronic active hepatitis, hepatic lipidosis, cholangitis, cholangiohepatitis, patients receiving drugs with hepatotoxic potential, and patients with decreased hepatobiliary function. Both S-adenosylmethionine (SAMe) and the silymarin complexes have proven to both be beneficial and therefore nutraceuticals that contain both ingredients should be sought.

S-Adenosylmethione

Glutathione is a major antioxidant produced by the liver; its main function is to reduce oxidative damage to the hepatocytes by free radicals. When the liver is compromised there is an increased production of free radicals, and thus the extent of the oxidative stress suffered by hepatocytes is increased. Thus an increased supply of glutathione is required as production is also decreased during hepatic disease. The supply of glutathione is via SAMe. SAMe initiates three major biochemical pathways: transmethylation, transulphuration and aminopropylation, which all help promote liver health and preserve functioning liver tissue. SAMe is found endogenously (within the body), being synthesised by the body's cells, including hepatocytes. SAMe is derived from ATP and methionine, and it initiates biochemical pathways involved in critical functions such as detoxification; modulating steroid hormone effects; cellular function and intracellular communication; regulating the Na^+/K^+-ATPase pump; and protecting cellular DNA. SAMe also has other important roles including cytoprotection, modulating inflammation, promoting cell replication, and protein synthesis and improving hepatocellular function.

Milk thistle

Milk thistle is a herb belonging to the genus *Silybum*, which contains an active antioxidant bioflavonoid complex known as silymarin. Silymarin stimulates the production of glutathione and glutathione perioxidase (see Chapter 13), and has cell-protective properties, especially within the liver. Silybin is the major active ingredient in silymarin, and has anti-inflammatory activity supporting hepatocyte regeneration, enhances bile flow and production of hepatoprotective bile salts, and increases gluthathione levels. Unlike SAMe, silybin is not naturally produced by liver cells and therefore an external nutritional source is required.

Key points

- Aid the client in any nutritional recommendations, dietary transitions, and general dietary advice.

- Discuss the use of supplements that aid hepatic function, SAMe, antioxidants, and the difference between veterinary-grade products and those found in health food shops.
- Monitor body weight and body condition score (BCS).
- Perform any diagnostic blood sampling required by the veterinary surgeon, also to aid the client in understanding the importance of routine screening.

29 Obesity

The nature of the veterinary profession is moving towards preventive/prophylaxis care rather than emergency medicine. Obesity has to be viewed as one of the many diseases that can be prevented, rather than having to be dealt with at the treatment stage.

Nurse clinics

The aims of nursing clinics and nutritional management diet to promote weight loss include:

- Supplying adequate nutrients, within a reduced-calorie diet.
- Promoting smooth weight loss, while maintaining a lean body mass as much as possible.
- Increasing conversion of stored fat to energy.
- Motivating the client to continue with the weight loss programme.
- Educating the client about potential behavioural traits that need to be altered in both the pet and the owner.

Prevention is obviously better than cure and the ideal place to start is in puppy clinics, first vaccinations and puppy parties. It has been clearly demonstrated that animals that remain at or marginally below their ideal weight throughout their growth phase are less likely to become obese in later life. Following-up puppies or kittens after neutering is vital. With a decrease in metabolism and change in diet many animals tend to increase their weight and body condition score (BCS) at this stage in life, and subsequently battle with it into adulthood. The veterinary nurse is the ideal person to discuss postoperative changes in diet and feeding amounts. Why not encourage all owner to bring their pets to see a veterinary nurse at 9 months of age, for a weight check (most animals will require worming at this stage to), and to discuss diet/feeding. Many animals are about to transition to a junior or adult light/neutered diet at this stage.

The Consulting Veterinary Nurse, First Edition. Nicola Ackerman.
© 2012 John Wiley & Sons, Ltd. Published 2012 by John Wiley & Sons, Ltd.

Owner education

Owners' perception of their animal's weight can vary, as it does with their own weight. Owners need to be advised/educated to what is deemed as obese or overweight. Management systems/protocols need to be in place in veterinary practices in order to aid in obesity prevention. Every animal should be weighed and recorded on each visit. The animal's weight can then be tracked throughout its life. It is also easier to estimate an ideal body weight for the animal if you know its weight and BCS history. It is also useful to be able to tell an owner, especially when you are seeing the animal through adolescence to adulthood, 'this is your pet's ideal weight'. Ensure that you log this in the clinical history. If the animal subsequently gains weight you can look back and say to the owner, 'Do you remember when your pet was this weight, and remember how active they were then?'.

Obesity is the most prevalent form of malnutrition in pets presented to veterinary practices. Obesity is defined as having body fat exceeding 15–20% of body weight (Debraekaleer 2004). Excessive weight is an associative cause or exacerbating factor for specific orthopaedic, endocrine, cardiovascular and neoplastic disease (Biourge 2001). Obesity will also make the animal less tolerant or resilient to metabolic stress (Figure 29.1). The weight and volume of fat in the abdomen of an obese animal can exert enough pressure on the bladder to induce leakage of urine, but also to reduce the diameter of the urethra and cause reduced flow of urine. The animal ultimately needs to change from a positive energy balance to a negative energy balance in order to lose and then maintain an ideal body weight.

Weight loss is an exceptionally difficult thing to achieve, and it is not just nutritional advice that is required in order to achieve this goal. Behavioural modifications of both the owner and pet are required, alongside advice on exercise – which can be difficult if the animal or owner has a mobility problem. In many cases owners are not receptive to comments that their pets are overweight, and it can

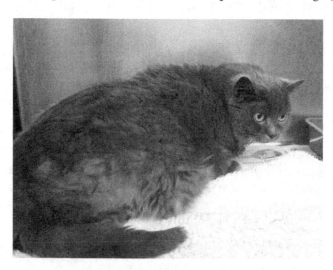

Figure 29.1 Obese cat.

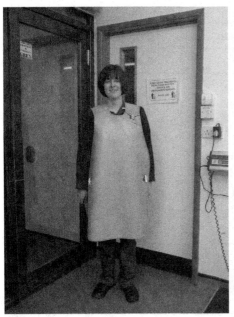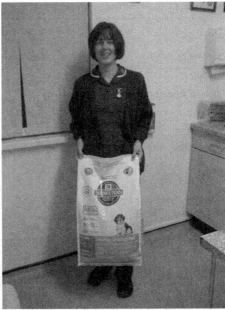

Figure 29.2 Practical demonstration of excessive weight gain is advantageous.

be really difficult to motivate owners to initiate a weight loss programme if they do not feel that there is a problem there initially. Some owners feel that being overweight by a few kilograms does not make any significant difference to the animal. The effect of being overweight can be easily demonstrated to an owner by asking them to put on the practice's lead radiography apron (Figure 29.2). This will demonstrate to the client that only a small amount of weight gain can be a significant percentage gain for the animal, depending on the animal's size.

Clinical nutrition

Satiation is related to the rate of food consumption (an animals can overeat before realising that it is satiated), food constituents (protein is more satiating than carbohydrates) and the animal's sense of fullness. These three factors should be used in the construction of a dietary plan in obesity control. Nutritional management is only part of a weight loss management programme; the animal's exercise levels and lifestyle also need to be considered.

Protein

Diets with high protein levels can be classed as low-energy diets, in comparison to those that are high in carbohydrates (Table 29.1). These diets can be advantageous as they conserve lean body mass while being efficient in inducing weight

Table 29.1 Calorific value of nutrients

	1 g carbohydrate	1 g protein	1 g fat
Gross energy	**4.2 kcal**	**5.4 kcal**	**9.4 kcal**
Gross energy → digestible energy			
	3.7 kcal	4.8 kcal	8.5 kcal
	88%	89%	90%
Digestible energy → metabolised energy			
	3.5 kcal	3.5 kcal	8.5 kcal
	83%	65%	90%
Metabolised energy → net energy			
True energy value	3.2 kcal	2.2 kcal	8.2 kcal
% of gross energy	76%	41%	87%

loss in cats. Values stated as kilocalories per gram are usually of metabolised energy and not the net energy gained by the diet. By using the net energy fraction, calorie differences are greater. This highlights the advantages of using a high-protein diet in cats (Martin 2001).

Carbohydrates

The role of carbohydrates in an obesity diet can be vital. Obesity diets can work by altering the levels of non-fermentable fibres. The role of the fibre is to achieve a sensation of satiety in the animal, while the providing a reduced proportion of calories within its diet. In some high-fibre obesity diets this can mean that only 60–70% of the animal's daily calorific requirement is obtained from the diet; the other 30–40% is obtained by utilising the animal's bodily fat reserves. High-fibre diets in cats may affect object play, and therefore reduce calorie expenditure, thus an exercise regime as part of a calorie-controlled diet is important to help retain the lean body mass.

This high level of fibre can have its disadvantages, including increased faecal output and possibly flatulence. This should be clearly explained to the owner if the weight loss plan is to be successful.

Fats

The fat level in an obesity diet needs to be restricted, in order to control calorific intake, but the diet must contain the necessary levels of essential fatty acids (EFA). Some obesity diets aid in weight loss by only providing the animal with about

60–70% of their daily energy requirements. The required energy shortfall is met by utilisation of the animal's body fat stores.

Vitamins and minerals

The oxidative cell damaged caused by free radicals is greater in obese animals. It is therefore recommended that the diet be supplemented with antioxidants (see Chapter 13). If comparing diets on a calorific value, vitamin and mineral levels in these diets will seem higher. This is due to the low-calorie nature of the diet. When comparing nutrient levels in these diets it is advisable to use other quantitative values. The typical vitamin and mineral values should be sufficient for the life stage of that particular individual.

L-Carnitine

L-Carnitine is a small, water-soluble, vitamin-like molecule (Pion 2004), which is concentrated in mammalian cardiac and skeletal muscle by an active membrane transport mechanism. It has been shown to increase body fat loss and prevent loss of muscle mass (Armstrong et al. 1992), and can also protect cats from hepatic lipid accumulation during calorie restriction (Gross et al. 1998). Most veterinary-grade obesity diets contain supplemented levels of L-carnitine.

Feeding an obesity diet

Weight reduction programmes initiated within the veterinary practice tend to be more successful, mainly due to close monitoring and the support offered. Programmes include three important stages:

1   A feeding plan, based on the amount of excess fat to lose and what is currently being fed
2   An exercise plan, based on mobility allowances and the owner's lifestyle and work commitments
3   A recheck plan.

Reduced calorie intake alone will not substantially reduce weight. For the weight reduction to be a success all three stages of the programme must be completed. Stage 3, the recheck plan, will depend on the case history, success of weight loss and the practice policy. In many cases a recheck every 2 weeks is normal.

In order to design a feeding plan correctly, the ideal body weight of the animal needs to be obtained. An ideal or optimal body weight should be calculated by examining the animal. Using body condition score (BCS) is the preferred way to assess the animal as it takes into account the animal's frame size independent of its weight. The animal's coat can also prove to be quite deceptive in obscuring whether it is underweight or overweight. Dogs and cats that have an optimal BCS have normal body contours; the bony prominences readily can be palpated under the skin surfaces. Looking back over the animal's previous weight history can aid in identifying the ideal body weight. If the animal had an ideal body condition score earlier in its life you can use this, or if the owner states that at 1 year of age the animal was at its ideal body weight this can be used. Once an ideal body weight has been calculated the amount of weight to be lost is now known.

Some therapeutic or prescription diets require the animal to be fed a set amount depending on the ideal body weight and adjusted thereafter from this quantity in 10% increments. Evaluating the animal's current diet and removing all titbits and snacks will aid in an initial loss of weight. This strategy will cause limited weight loss in most animals. Reduction in quantities of a maintenance diets can lead to deficiencies in important nutrients, and should be avoided.

All weight loss diets have their advantages and disadvantages, and any disadvantages of using high-fibre diets should be explained to the owners. If owners are not forewarned about increases in defecation and faecal output, this can cause them to cease feeding the diet. Encouraging the owner to feed the last daily diet earlier, and giving the animal either more access to the litter tray or the ability to go outside, will eliminate any problems. The correct ratio is to feed 60–70% of the maintenance rate for the animal's body weight. Fat will then be utilised to make up the shortfall.

Once the ideal weight has been achieved, maintaining this optimal weight can be difficult, and even more frequent weight check-ups may be required. Owner encouragement is still recommended to keep up established exercise regimes and positive feeding habits, as lost weight can easily be regained. Dog and cats will experience a 'rebound' effect after weight loss if fed an uncontrolled diet (LaFlamme and Kuhlman 1993). Selection of a new diet once the optimal weight has been achieved can be difficult, and can vary from animal to animal. Some will maintain the optimal weight well on a light life stage diet, combined with an exercise programme. Others will require a modified amount of the obesity diet or a transitional therapeutic weight control diet.

The length of time required to reach optimal weight depends on the individual patient. It can be calculated as follows:

$$\frac{\text{initial bwt (g)} - \text{target bwt (g)}}{\text{weekly weight loss (g)}} = \text{time to reach target bwt (weeks)}$$

The weekly weight loss can differ from week to week, especially in cats, whose activity levels can vary greatly, and usually depend on the weather. In multi-cat households there is often one fat cat and one or more lean cats. Play and activity feeding should be emphasised. Tunnels or small holes, which the fat cat cannot get through, can be utilised to allow feeding access for the leaner cats.

Behaviour and its role in obesity

Cats

Behaviour plays an important role in obesity and should be addressed with the owner. This involves behavioural interactions between other animals in the household and between the owner and the animal. Cats can easily become obese in a multi-cat household due to overeating. In these situations cats need to have their own, safe, feeding station. Each feeding station needs be separate from the litter tray and from the cat's own water bowl. There need to be more water bowls and feeding bowls than there are cats in the household, all of them in different positions.

In most cases the obese cat in the multi-cat household is the most nervous one. Cat behaviour is very difficult for owners to interpret, and many do not perceive that there is a tension in the air between their own cats. Cats can be known to binge eat when other cats are not present near the feeding bowl. Owners can interpret this as the obese cat not eating much, as it only goes to the bowl very infrequently, normally when the owners are not there, and eats very fast. This can result in the overall intake being taken higher than normal. In these cases it can be useful to have a 'safe room' in the house for the nervous cat, which can be feed separately away from the others and eat at its own pace. This feeding regime can also be utilised for cats suffering from FLUTD, as the reduction in stress can help to prevent reoccurrence.

Cats have adapted to eat little and often, and changing a cat to meal-based feeding can be difficult. Owners should be encouraged to weigh out the daily rations of food on weighing scales. This allocated amount of diet can then be used throughout the day to feed the cat little and often. Encouraging the cat to exercise is always recommended; throwing single kibbles for the cat to eat will encourage movement. The use of light beams is also beneficial, but after the cat has chased the light around, the light should always end on a toy that the cat can pounce on and attack. This satisfies the cat's hunting behaviour, and will prevent the it becoming frustrated with the play behaviour. Discuss with the owner that the cat's behaviour is not normal – lying around the house all day and night is not normal for a cat.

Dogs

The main behavioural element relevant to obesity in dogs is the giving and receiving of treats. Weight loss is not just about nutrition and exercise regimes. It is mainly about human psychology, as veterinary nurse who runs clinics will tell you this. Feeding = love, and it is an opportunity to interact and exchange affection and touch; it is deemed a fun activity by owners. We all know that dieting is not fun, and owners perceive this in their pets, hungry means unhappy, which equates to losing love. If dieting were easy, we would all be slim; but it is not, it is difficult. Dieting requires changing habits, which can be uncomfortable and hard. Internally the owner requires motivation, but externally support is also required – the ideal role for the veterinary nurse.

Pharmaceuticals

The use of pharmaceuticals can also affect canine behaviour. While not entirely understood, the proposed mechanisms of microsomal triglyceride transfer protein (MTP) inhibitors in weight loss include both inhibition of dietary lipid absorption across the intestine and stimulation of gut hormones that signal satiety, e.g. glucagon-like peptide 1 (GLP-1) and peptide YY (PYY). The use of pharmaceuticals can be helpful for those owners who find it difficult to cope with begging behaviour from their dogs. Potential problems can arise when owners feel that their pets no longer love them, as the dog is not greeting them at the door when they come home from work. Owners mistake this behaviour as a welcome home, rather than the dog looking for a food source. When a food-orientated dog has the drive for food removed it will alter its behaviour greatly. Owners should be informed of these possible changes.

Rewards for the dog need to be altered from food to another form of reward. Interactions from the owner have tended to be the handing over a treat, and then the dog goes back to whatever it was doing beforehand. Encouraging the owner to play with the dog, groom the dog or take the dog out for a walk are all different methods of interaction that the owner can undertake. Ongoing weight management is required, as discontinuation of the drugs results in return of appetite and weight gain if food intake is not controlled.

During the period that the dog is receiving the pharmaceuticals any undesired behaviours associated with food – not only of the dog but also of the owner –need to be addressed.

Tips for obesity clinics

Establishing a successful obesity clinic in your practice is a major priority in order to help treat this major problem. The dietary regime for weight loss should not just be considered an option, but rather as a medical treatment of obesity.

Before you can set up a weight loss clinic several points need to be clarified. These include length of appointments, what food is to be recommended, if any, how often you want to see the pet, and the charging policy charge for any nurse clinics dealing with obesity.

It is easy to prescribe a diet, work out the amounts of food needed, and the amount of exercise that the animal requires. The greatest difficulty of any weight loss clinic is motivating the owner (see Box 29.1).

Box 29.1   Obesity clinic protocol

1   At the initial consultation, weigh the animal and assess body condition score (BCS). A decision needs to be made on which version of BCS you want to use, as the same one needs to be used throughout. Record the weight and BCS on animal's clinical history. A checklist and weight loss graph can be used, and many of the pet food manufacturers can provide these. This will ensure that a complete feeding history is taken. Take 'before' photo. The initial consult usually takes 30–40 minutes. Appendix 1 shows an example of a feeding history sheet.

2   Once all the facts have been obtained, dietary modifications need to be made. This can include change of diet, feeding quantities, titbits, dental chews. Obesity medication needs to be authorised by a veterinary surgeon, and can aid with behavioural traits associated with obesity loss.

3   Depending on whether the owner wishes to use a prescription diet or keep to a life stage diet, set amounts of food and exercise, and establish reweigh programmes.

4   Design an exercise regime for the pet. Small frequent, periods of exercise are more beneficial than one longer walk. Many obese animals have extremely low exercise tolerance. Hydrotherapy should only be recommended once exercise tolerance has increased, as it is very demanding cardiovascularly.

5   At the first consultation, give the client your business card, in case they need to contact the practice. Having a designated point of contact can help increase compliance with the weight loss programme (see Chapter 6).

6   Two days after the first consultation, contact the owner to find out how they are coping. Are they complying with the dietary, exercise and behavioural changes that have been introduced? Follow up with further phone call if required.

7   On first reweigh, reassess feeding quantities dependent on weight gain or loss.

8   Reweigh every 2 weeks until you are happy that the animal is losing weight well. The animal can then be weighed every month until the target weight reached. (Phone contact every 2 weeks is still advised in order to help with compliance.)

9   If the animal is not losing weight well, reduce the food amount by 10%. More importantly, the exercise levels need to be increased.

10 Exercise levels can be increased by more walks. For an animal that is arthritic or has poor exercise intolerance, an increase in frequency rather than length is more beneficial to the animal. For dogs, swimming, and searching for food with the use of food balls can be instigated. For cats, food balls can also be used; also positioning the food so that they have to move around to get it, and the use of lasers/toys to make them play/exercise.

11 If the animal is not happy on a specific diet, don't be afraid to use a different brand. The brand of diet to be used should be the one that benefits the patient and owner the most, not the one that the practice stocks.

Tips for weight loss

It can be useful to have a printed list of top tips to give to the owner when starting out on the weight loss programme. There will mostly reiterate what has already been covered during the course of the obesity clinic, but they aid in the compliance of the owner to attend clinics.

- Have regular weight checks with a pet slimmer's clinic/nurse. Regular contact with the pet slimmer's nurse can dramatically help with your pet's weight loss. Feeding quantities may need adjusting in order to find the correct amount for your pet.

- Weigh out the daily food allowance in the morning, put it in a container, and use this food for the allocated meals. This way you are less likely to overfeed. You can take out a few kibbles to use as treats throughout the day.
- Increase exercise levels gently. It is important for the pet slimmer's nurse to help design an exercise programme. Little and often can prove to be more beneficial for weight loss. Cats can exercise by use of toys, light torches, etc., but always ensure that this play activity ends on an object. This will satisfy the cat's hunting activities, and they won't get frustrated.
- Placing the food in different areas or hiding kibbles around the house/room can encourage cats to exercise more. Use of a food ball is ideal in these situations.
- If you have more than one cat, it important to feed them separately, and to observe them when they are eating.
- It can be wise to inform your neighbours that your pet is going on a weight loss programme, and ask them not to feed it.
- For a weight loss programme to be successful everyone involved in caring for the pet, or who may feed the pet, needs to be involved and 'on board'.
- It is important that no 'extras' are added to your pet's daily allocated allowance. This also includes milk and cat milk.

Obesity in rabbits

See Chapter 14.

Key points

- Communication with the owner about feeding and exercise regimes is vital if weight loss is to occur.
- All relevant factors, e.g. exercise regime, number of pets in the household, etc., must be considered if successful weight loss is to happen.
- Behaviour is an extremely important part of weight loss, and attention should be given to this subject, and its effect on weight loss.

References

Armstrong PJ, Hardie EM, Cullen JM. L-Carnitine reduces hepatic fat accumulation during rapid weight reduction in cats. *Proc 10th Vet Med Forum* 1992; 810.

Biourge V. Obesity, a major risk factor for diabetes in cats. In: *Royal Canin's Guide to Feline Obesity*. Royal Canin Publications 2001, pp. 10–13.

Debraekaleer J. Obesity in cats and dogs. *Vet Times* 2004; 22 March:14.

Gross KL, Wedekind KJ, Kirk CA. Effect of dietary carnitine or chromium on weight loss and body composition of obese dogs. *J Anim Sci* 1998;76 suppl 1: 175.

LaFlamme DP, Kuhlman G. The effect of weight loss on subsequent weight maintenance in dogs. *J Vet Inter Med* 1993; 7:134.

Martin L. The principle of high-protein diets and net energy. In: *Royal Canin's Guide to Feline Obesity*. Royal Canin Publications 2001, pp. 6–9.

Pion PD. Traditional and nontraditional effective and noneffective therapies for cardiac disease in dogs and cats. *Vet Clin North Am Small Anim Pract* 2004; 34:187–216.

30 Pancreatic Disorders

Exocrine pancreatic insufficiency

Exocrine pancreatic insufficiency (EPI) describes a lack of pancreatic enzymes (lipase and amylase) in the gut lumen, resulting in steatorrhoea and weight loss. When lipases are absent from the array of brush border enzymes, secondary damage to the small intestine and small intestinal bacterial overgrowth (SIBO) can occur. These complications can further aggravate the malabsorption of nutrients. EPI occurs commonly in young dogs as a congenital abnormality, but may also develop as a sequela to acute or chronic pancreatitis. EPI is rare in cats, but has been reported in both the juvenile and acquired forms.

Nurse clinic

The animal will be referred to a nurse clinic once it has been diagnosed with EPI. The aims of the nurse clinic are to:

- Help the client with the understanding of the diagnosis, and what this means for long-term treatment regimes
- Provide regular weight checks and body condition scores (BCS).

The role of nutritional management includes:

- Providing a highly digestible diet.
- Supplementation of exocrine pancreatic enzymes in each meal

The diet needs to provide sufficient calories and nutrients to support the particular life stage of the animal. This may have to be higher than calculated due to the changes in digestion and metabolism.

The Consulting Veterinary Nurse, First Edition. Nicola Ackerman.
© 2012 John Wiley & Sons, Ltd. Published 2012 by John Wiley & Sons, Ltd.

Clinical nutrition

Fat

Effective treatment of EPI involves the supplementation of pancreatic enzyme. There are many preparations available on the market, the most effective being in the form of powders that can be sprinkled onto the diet prior to ingestion. A low-fat, highly digestible diet is recommended as a starting point in EPI and is particularly valuable if there is persistent SIBO. The dry matter digestibility of these diets needs to be greater than 90%.

Once the dog has reached its optimal weight and condition there is no reason why it should not return to a good-quality life stage diet, with the addition of the pancreatic enzymes. Some larger dogs may find it difficult to achieve a high enough calorific intake on a low-fat diet.

Carbohydrates

Soluble fibre in the diet is important in order to help resolve SIBO, as it will help, to promote normalisation of the gastrointestinal flora. However. large amounts of fibre in the diet (especially insoluble fibre) will decrease the digestibility of the diet. The diet should contain no more than 2% fibre on a dry matter basis. The use of prebiotics in these cases can prove to be advantageous.

Proteins

Protein levels for animals suffering from EPI need to be adequate, as protein is utilised for energy metabolism if insufficient fat for this requirement is absorbed. If the diet has a good carbohydrate level, excessive protein quantities are not required; the amount should be appropriate for the particular life stage of the animal.

Vitamins and minerals

When any malassimilation or malabsorption is present, supplementation with micronutrients should be considered. When gastrointestinal fat absorption is impaired, so is the solubilisation and absorption of the fat-soluble vitamins. Vitamins A and D can be administered intramuscularly, and vitamin K should also be supplemented if coagulopathies are detected in the patient.

Folate and cobalamin/B_{12} levels are also of concern in the animal suffering from EPI. The absence of pancreatic bicarbonate secretion in EPI may reduce intestinal luminal pH and the affinity of cobalamin for intrinsic factor. If there is an overgrowth of luminal bacteria this gut microflora may consume the dietary cobalamin before it can be absorbed. Folate deficiencies have been shown to inhibit pancreatic exocrine function in rats, and therefore if any deficiencies are present, supplementation with parenteral folate is recommended.

Feeding an animal with EPI

On diagnosis of EPI an initial transition to a highly digestible, low-fat diet is beneficial. This will aid in the normalisation of the gut transit times, absorption of nutrients and gastrointestinal flora. Daily administration of pre- and probiotics will also aid in the re-establishment of normal gastrointestinal flora populations. Dogs presenting with EPI always tend to be underweight, and assessment of weight gain needs to be monitored.

Even after the animal has reached its ideal body weight, it may be necessary to offer the calculated basal energy requirement (BER) plus 20% to allow for the persistent degree of malabsorption in patients with EPI.

Supplements

All patients with EPI should be fed multiple small meals per day, with pancreatic enzyme supplementation in order to improve digestibility, dietary overload and osmotic diarrhoea. It is more beneficial for the enzyme supplements to be added to the diet at least 5 minutes prior to consumption. Capsules should always be opened and sprinkled over the diet for each meal.

Pancreatitis

The exocrine pancreas is highly responsive to changes in nutritional substrates present within the diet. When the pancreas becomes inflamed, symptoms such as depression, anorexia, vomiting, diarrhoea and signs of abdominal pain can present. Pancreatitis, whether acute or chronic, is commonly seen in veterinary practice. It is exceptionally painful, because the proteolytic enzymes are activated *in situ* resulting in autodigestion, and requires analgesia as its primary treatment. There are many factors that can predispose to pancreatitis, including breed, age, gender, neuter status and body condition.

Nurse clinic

The nurse clinic plays an important role in the management of patients with pancreatitis. There are many different aspects of management with these patients, and owners will need support.

Treatment of pancreatitis involves consideration of the following factors:

- Treatment/removal of the initial cause.
- Fluid therapy, in order to maintain hydration and electrolyte levels; plasma may be required in severe cases.
- Analgesia. Non-steroidal anti-inflammatory drugs (NSAIDs) are best avoided in these cases due to the gastric and renal side effects. Non-ulcerogenic NSAIDs could be considered in chronic cases.

- Nutritional status of the animal. On a short-term basis should the animal be starved, tube fed, or given total parenteral nutrition (TPN)? There is current conflicting evidence to support each. Thoughts should also be given to long-term dietary management.
- Symptomatic treatment with antiemetics, antibiotics and antiulcer medication as necessary to prevent complications. The use of broad-spectrum antibiotics serves a dual purpose: first to combat any infection that might be present, and secondly to protect against septicaemia caused by bacterial translocation.
- In cats hyperglycaemia is often noted, but can be mild and transient; however, in some cases diabetes mellitus can develop and may require insulin therapy.

The aims of clinical nutrition in these cases are really important and are the mainstay of management of these cases:

- To provide sufficient calories and nutrients to the body without overloading the pancreas
- Preventing the possibility of bacterial translocation from the gastrointestinal tract and intestinal atrophy.

Clinical nutrition

Fat

Fat in the diet delays gastric emptying, which can in turn promote vomiting in the dog or cat. The delay in gastric emptying is a significant cause of upper gastrointestinal signs in the dog, including abdominal discomfort, nausea and vomiting. Preventing or inhibiting the release of pancreatic enzymes that aid in digestion of fats is an essential component of treatment. For long-term management, feeding a low-fat diet with or without the use of pancreatic enzymes can reduce postprandial pain. Restricting the fat content of the diet is not as vital in cats as in dogs, but the diet should still be of a highly digestible nature.

Carbohydrates

As the fat content in the diet needs to be reduced yet highly digestible, the carbohydrate content must provide a greater contribution to the metabolisable energy (ME) content of the diet. The carbohydrates present in the diet must be easily digestible, as digestion and absorption may be adversely affected in all cases of gastrointestinal upset.

Vitamins and minerals

Guidelines for vitamin and mineral levels are the same as for that particular life stage. Care should be taken if large volumes of vomiting or diarrhoea are present, as excessive amounts of the water-soluble vitamins can be lost. When feeding an exceptionally low-fat diet, the quantity of fat-soluble vitamins can also be lost. As some of these vitamins are required in fat metabolism it is important that these losses are replaced.

Hypokalaemia is particularly common in animals suffering from pancreatitis, and can be severe and life threatening. If vomiting or diarrhoea is present then electrolyte balance must be monitored, as it should be with any animal receiving intravenous fluid therapy. Oral supplementation may be required.

Supplements

The use of exocrine pancreatic enzymes in cases of acute pancreatitis is now becoming commonplace in veterinary practice. Even if the animal is not displaying clinical symptoms of EPI, these enzymes have an important part to play. Addition of the enzymes to the meal at least 5 minutes before feeding has been proven to reduce postprandial pain, and helps to ease the pancreas back into work after a period of 'rest'.

Feeding a pancreatic patient

Current dietary therapy for dogs suffering from acute pancreatitis is nil-by-mouth, until the clinical symptoms stop, and in some practices this can be up to 5–7 days. Recent evidence has shown that nil-by-mouth in these cases has little benefit to the animal. In acute pancreatic cases, withholding food is only indicated when the animal is vomiting. Any cases requiring this for more than 24 hours TPN must be provided, alongside very small amounts of nutrition being given by mouth (micro-enteral nutrition). The oral nutritional support is required to prevent gastroduo-denal ulceration, bacterial translocation from the gut and septicaemia. Small amounts of watered-down baby rice or cottage cheese can be used before moving onto a commercial low-fat, highly digestible diet. Baby rice is the food of choice in these cases; a typical nutrient analysis is shown in Table 27.3.

In cats, nutrition is generally supplied by enteral means (gastrostomy feeding tube), in order to avoid hepatic lipidosis. There is no clinical evidence that this type of nutrition exacerbates the course of acute pancreatitis. There is also evidence that enteral support is superior to parenteral support as described as above. Oral intake in cats should only be restricted if persistent vomiting is occurring, and then for as short a time as possible.

Dietary long-term control of pancreatitis is vital, but initially the presence of hyperlipidaemia needs to be confirmed. Dogs suffering from pancreatitis with associated hyperlipidaemia will need to be maintained on a different diet from those without. If the lipid levels in the bloodstream are within normal levels, then a highly digestible low-fat diet can be used. If hyperlipidaemia is concurrent then a low-fat diet is also required, but these types of diets can have a correspondingly high fibre content, thus reducing digestibility. This can be advantageous, as the majority of dogs that suffer from hyperlipidaemia tend to be overweight and can benefit from this type of diet anyway.

Weight control is important in these cases, as a major predisposing factor is obesity and being fed high-fat treats. By altering the diet in order to reduce fat content, most animals will gradually lose weight, but this does need to be monitored regularly.

Key points

- Analgesia: this is the most important aspect of treating any animal with pancreatitis.
- Use of minimal enteral nutrition in order to prevent bacterial translocation.
- Use of exogenous pancreatic enzymes.

31 Renal Disorders

In all animals, clinical symptoms of renal dysfunction are not evident until 65–75% of renal tissue has been destroyed. Many veterinary practices instigate renal screening for older patients and before starting of pharmaceutical regimes. Nutritional management can affect many consequences of renal failure, and is the cornerstone of management. Chronic renal failure (CRF) has many physiological effects: these include the decreased ability to excrete nitrogenous waste (and thus build-up of azotaemia), sodium and phosphorus, and an increased loss of potassium. Other clinical symptoms also include systemic hypertension, secondary hyperparathyroidism and non-regenerative anaemia, and should be monitored as part of the nursing clinic (Lane 2005).

Nurse clinic

Nurse clinics for animals that have newly diagnosed or suspected renal disease should be instigated as soon as possible. All patients should be referred to the nurse, in order to discuss diet, medications (if required), compliance and any future requirements for diagnostics and reviews of the patient. The nurse is also well placed to answer any questions that the owner may have.

Aims of nurse clinic

The aim of the nurse clinic for renal patients is to aid the client:

- In the preservation of the remaining renal tissue
- To reduce accumulation of nitrogenous waste in the blood stream by minimising protein precursors for urea
- To correct fluid, electrolyte and acid–base balance
- To provide adequate calories to prevent further catabolism or malnutrition, helping to maintain an ideal body condition score (BCS)

The Consulting Veterinary Nurse, First Edition. Nicola Ackerman.
© 2012 John Wiley & Sons, Ltd. Published 2012 by John Wiley & Sons, Ltd.

- To ensure compliance of the owner with medications, if any, and repeat diagnostic monitoring methods
- To ensure that the animal's blood pressure is controlled, by routine monitoring and referral back to the veterinary surgeon as required
- To provide support to the client during the later stages of the animal's life.

Diagnostic monitoring

The International Renal Interest Society (IRIS) have developed a renal scoring index that helps to identify the progression of the disease in order to facilitate appropriate treatment and monitoring of the patient. The initial staging is based on a fasted plasma creatinine level, and then sub-staged dependent on proteinuria levels and arterial blood pressure (Table 31.1). Fasted blood samples must always be used, as even a moderately high protein meal prior to sampling can elevate blood plasma creatinine levels. Repeat blood sampling should be done as required, but should be performed more regularly if urinalysis shows changes in proteinuria levels.

Owners may need guidance on methods on how to obtain urine samples, as these are the most useful diagnostic tools in the progression of renal failure. Urine concentration should be routinely measured by a refractometer, and the urine protein creatinine (UP/C) ratio (Table 31.2) should be routinely assessed.

Table 31.1   IRIS recommendation of renal staging based on plasma creatinine levels

Plasma creatinine level (µmol/L)	Stage 1	Stage 2	Stage 3	Stage 4
Dog	<125	125–179	180–439	440+
Cat	<140	140–249	250–439	440+
Maintain phosphate within specific ranges in relation to stage:				
Serum phosphate target (mmol/L)	N/A	0.81–1.45	0.81–1.61	0.81–1.94
Action	Not required	Renal diet or phosphate binder	Renal diet ± phosphate binder	

Reproduced with permission from Novartis Animal Health Inc.

Table 31.2   Urine protein/creatinine (UP/C) ratio

	Cats	Dogs
Non-proteinuric	<0.2	<0.2
Borderline	0.2–0.4	0.2–0.5
Proteinuric	>0.4	>0.5

Reproduced with permission from Novartis Animal Health Inc.

Table 31.3 Substaging renal failure with blood pressure monitoring

Systolic BP (mmHg)	Diastolic BP (mmHg)	Adaptation when breed specific reference range is available	Arterial pressure substage	Risk
<150	<95	<10 mmHg above reference range	0	Minimal
150–159	95–99	10–20 mmHg above reference range	1	Low
160–179	100–119	20–40 mmHg above reference range	2	Moderate
≥180	≥120	≥40 mmHg above reference range	3	High

BP, blood pressure.
Adapted by IRIS. Reproduced with permission from Novartis Animal Health Inc.

Medications such as angiotensin converting enzyme (ACE) inhibitors should only be instigated when proteinuria is present. It should be noted that proteinuria can present at any stage of the renal failure, and is not directly linked to the level of azotaemia.

All newly diagnosed renal patients should have their blood pressure monitored. Renal function is directly affected by an increase in blood pressure, and as the kidneys play a role in blood pressure secondary hypertension can result (Table 31.3). Hypertension should be treated, as its effects are ultimately negative.

Pharmaceuticals

The most commonly used pharmaceutical in animals with chronic renal failure is benazepril (POM-V), an ACE inhibitor. Inhibition of ACE leads to reduced conversion of inactive angiotensin I into active angiotensin II, therefore reducing the effects mediated by angiotensin II, including vasoconstriction of both arteries and veins, retention of sodium and water by the kidney, and modelling changes (including pathological cardiac hypertrophy and degenerative renal changes). In cats with chronic renal insufficiency benazepril reduces the protein loss in urine and reduces systemic and intraglomerular blood pressure; it also helps to increase appetite, quality of life and survival time, particularly in advanced disease. Benazepril is therefore indicated when proteinuria is present, and this should therefore be tested for. As ACE inhibitors decrease the intraglomerular blood pressure there will be a refractory increase in nitrogenous waste products.

In some cases addition hypertensive medications may be required in order to return the patient to a normotensive state. In these cases amlodipine (POM) may be added into the regime. Once this is instigated, blood pressure monitoring is required in order to taper the dose according to the patient's readings.

If medications are prescribed for patients with CRF it is important that the veterinary nurse discusses with the client attending the clinic whether they are able to medicate their pet. Owners may need guidance on the administration of medications.

Clinical nutrition

The role of diet is very important in aiding in the longevity and quality of life of the animal. As many animals are azotaemic it can be very difficult to instigate dietary changes. By understanding the ideal nutrient requirements for an animal with renal failure, guidance can be offered when owners wish to prepare home-made diets or feed a commercial diet.

Water

Renal disease causes a progressive decline in urine-concentrating capacity. Dehydration, volume depletion, renal hypoperfusion and dietary salt intake stimulate urine concentration. Avoiding dehydration and renal hypoperfusion reduces the work of concentrating the urine and helps to maintain intrarenal protective mechanisms. Patients with CRF must have unlimited access to fresh water and free choice consumption. This can be exceptionally important in cats, which have fastidious drinking habits.

Increasing water consumption can be achieved in a number of different ways (see Chapter 12). Feeding a moist diet rather than a dry diet, and increasing the availability of water by placing more bowls around the house and in the garden, will aid in increasing water consumption. Allowing water to stand for a period of time before offering it to some animals can be beneficial. This allows the chlorine in the water to evaporate off, which some animals prefer.

Protein

The majority of veterinary diets for dogs are in two 'phases', indicated for the different stages of CRF. This staged management system is recommended in dogs, as early cases can benefit from phosphorus restriction, while maintaining a protein intake level equal to an adult maintenance level. Early cases are defined as those that are azotaemic and not uraemic, and make up 18–20% of dogs suffering from CRF.

For dogs that are presented with uraemia, the diet needs to have a lower protein level. This will help to reduce the production of protein catabolites. The protein that is present in these diets needs to be of a high biological value to minimise the risk of essential amino acid deficiency. If protein is too restricted in either cats or dogs with CRF, hypoalbuminaemia, anaemia and metabolic acidosis can occur. It is therefore important to attain the correct balance of protein levels. If protein levels are too high, protein can act as a source of calories through deamination in the liver, and the nitrogenous waste products will then exacerbate the azotaemia.

Previous studies have implicated dietary protein as a direct possible causative, or a decrease in already dysfunctioning kidneys (Robertson et al. 1986). The majority of these studies were conducted with rats. Subsequently, studies have identified that the dog (and possibly cat, horse and rabbit), different from the rat in their response to dietary protein (Allen et al. 2000).

Proteinuria of glomerular origin was traditionally considered to be a consequence of damage to the glomerular barrier (Elliott 2005), but some studies have shown that proteinuria observed in association with an increased protein intake may be related to haemodynamic alteration and physiological changes in glomerular selectivity, rather than damage to the glomerular filtration barrier (Elliott 2005). An increase in protein excretion in urine is attributed to the passage of time (wear and tear) rather than protein and phosphorus levels (Elliott 2005), and underlines that urinalysis is a valuable, and often underutilised, diagnostic tool in detecting CRF and its severity.

The level of protein restriction is important in cats. Veterinary diets designed for renal management in cats do not have staged protein restriction levels. This is because cats cannot reduce the enzyme activity in their liver. These enzymes are involved in protein catabolism, and if the dietary protein level is greatly restricted, then protein malnutrition can occur. As with dogs, the protein level should be adequate for the animal's needs, but not so high so that excess is used as an energy source.

Vitamins and minerals

Sodium levels in renal diets are reduced. This is because of the reduction in the number of viable nephrons within the kidneys. As serum sodium levels remain the same, this means that each nephron has an increased load delivery. This, in turn, will create hypertension, as the blood pressure rises. Hence, blood pressure monitoring is recommended in animals with renal dysfunction. Sodium levels should not be too restricted, however, as this can result in a reduced capacity to reabsorb bicarbonate, which will contribute to metabolic acidosis. If sodium intake is rapidly reduced, dehydration and volume contraction may occur. A gradual change in diets is recommended when changing to a salt-restricted diet due to this, and a perceived decrease in palatability. Recommended sodium levels in renal diets are 0.3% (DMB) for cats and 0.2% (DMB) for dogs (Lane 2005).

Phosphorus is absorbed from the gastrointestinal tract, and primarily excreted by the kidneys. A restriction in dietary phosphorus has been shown to slow the progression of renal failure in cats and dogs. Hyperphosphataemia is a common finding in patients with CRF, and occurs when the glomerular filtration rate (GFR) falls below 20% of the norm. Consequently, this can result in reduced renal phosphate excretion, and hence raised serum levels. This can result in renal mineralisation and secondary hyperparathyroidism, thereby exacerbating renal damage, and aid in the development of hyperlipidaemia. If dietary means alone do not reduce serum phosphorus levels, then oral phosphorus-binding agents can be used. It has been shown that cats that have low phosphate levels in their diets live almost 2.5 times longer that cats that are fed normal diets (Elliott et al. 2000).

Potassium deficiency has been identified in cats with CRF (Plantinga et al. 2005). Hypokalaemia also impairs protein synthesis, promotes weight loss and a poor hair coat and contributes to polyuria by decreasing the renal responsiveness to antidiuretic hormone (ADH) (Elliott 2005).

Metabolic acidosis should be prevented, as it may be associated with increased ammoniagenesis and the progression of renal disease. If acidosis is present, an alkalinising agent should added. As sodium bicarbonate will increase sodium levels, either potassium or calcium carbonate can be used. Some veterinary diets adjust the levels of potassium in order to help prevent acidosis, but as each case is different, monitoring of the acid–base balance is recommended.

It is important to remember that with any disease or disorder that shows the clinical symptoms of polydipsia and polyuria, water-soluble vitamins can be lost. Water-soluble vitamin deficiency can further contribute to anorexia, as even higher demands are placed on these vitamins as the body tries to recuperate. Further supplementation with water-soluble vitamins is often not required, as commercially available veterinary diets contain additional quantities of these vitamins.

Fats

As discussed earlier, the renal patient needs to gain calories from a non-protein source. This can be from fats (lipids) or carbohydrates. The addition of fats to the diet is beneficial, as they provide twice as much energy per gram as carbohydrates and aid in palatability. The use of fatty acids has also been shown to decrease inflammation in the kidney, lower hypertension and preserve renal function. Veterinary diets are therefore supplemented with omega fatty acids or polyunsaturated fatty acids, especially eicosapentaenoic acid (EPA) and arachidonic acid (Plantinga et al. 2005). Omega-6 fatty acids appear to be detrimental in dogs with naturally occurring renal disease, by acutely increasing GFR.

Carbohydrates

Most manufacturers of veterinary diets do not realise the importance of dietary fibre in the management of renal disease. The animal itself cannot digest soluble fibre in the diet, but the microbes within the intestine can. Soluble fibre is fermented into short-chain fatty acids (SCFA) or volatile fatty acids (VFA). These products are an important energy source for the intestinal cells and can increase blood flow to the intestine.

Nitrogenous waste products in the blood are presented to the intestinal lumen where urease, an enzyme produced by intestinal bacteria, hydrolyses the urea into ammonia and carbon dioxide. The ammonia is then utilised by the intestinal bacteria. This process means that nitrogenous waste products are excreted in faecal matter, rather than in urine by the kidneys. Dietary fibre may also be beneficial for improving gastrointestinal motility in dogs with renal failure. Colonic transit times can be decreased in moderate renal disease as it alters duodenojejunal motility.

Supplements

Supplements that can be used in cases of chronic renal diseases are designed to help reduce the phosphate levels in the diet. Phosphate binders that can be used include calcium carbonate, which can reduce the apparent digestibility of phosphorus more than twofold compared to a standard diet.

Chitosan (a derivative of chitin) has also been used in supplements for animals suffering from chronic renal failure. Chitosan acts as an absorbent in the intestines, and thus lowers the absorption of certain substances including phosphates and some uraemic toxins.

A highly palatable formulation of medicinal rhubarb derived from the rhizome and roots of the rhubarb plant (*Rheum officinale*), which has been documented in tests with a variety of species to help protect healthy renal tissue, can also be used for cats with CRF. It helps to support normal renal functioning, which can be damaged by the cellular and enzymatic events occurring in renal injury through acute insult or persistent inflammation and the subsequent healing response. If untreated, this cascade of events can lead to fibrosis and related loss of glomerular filtration. One effective strategy in managing the disease is intervening at an early stage to minimise the negative consequences of fibrosis, and therefore there is a role for use of these supplements in the management of these cases.

Feeding a renal diet

Objectively, the role of these veterinary diets is to help reduce azotaemia, hyperphosphataemia, and also to control secondary hyperparathyroidism, ultimately improving both the clinical and biochemical status of the animal. But a reduced dietary intake has often been blamed on the palatability of the diet. The effect of uraemia on the sense of taste and smell and the development of food aversions can all contribute towards inappetance. Changing any animal from a high-salt, high-protein diet to a commercial renal diet can be very difficult. Changing via a transitional intermediate diet over a more prolonged period of time can be beneficial in these animals (see also information about feeding a low-salt diet on page 140).

The monitoring of animals with CRF by sampling both urine and blood is very important, and underutilised. Regular monitoring to ensure dietary and medical management remain optimal for each individual animal is vital for long-term successful management. Compliance from the owner can also be improved with this extra support from the veterinary practice. The disease processes should be monitored; this will include laboratory evaluation of blood and urine, blood pressure monitoring, full clinical history, physical examination, body weight and BCS. A history should also be taken of the amount of food and water being consumed. Owners find it difficult to differentiate between time spent at the food or water bowl and actual amount consumed; careful questioning may be necessary.

When initiating an animal on to a renal diet, a gradual transitional period is required. Gradual changes through a range of diets from adult to senior to early renal can be beneficial for animals more sensitive to the changes in salt content of the diet. They can also prove useful for owners with preconceptions about changing an animal from a supermarket high-salt brand to one of restricted salt and reduced protein levels. There is often a misconception that the palatability of renal diets is poor; in fact, the palatability of these diets is good. As most animals are accustomed to a higher salt level in their diet, changing to a lower-salt diet can cause difficulties, just as it does for people who are used to adding salt to their diets; their food tastes blander when they stop doing so. This is nothing to do with the diet itself; rather, the taste buds have to readjust to the reduction of salt in the food.

The decrease of protein levels in the diet results in a relative increase of the fat and carbohydrate levels. This results in an increase in calorific value and probable palatability due to the fat content. The increase in fat content can also cause digestive upsets such as diarrhoea. If the dietary transition has been made over a gradual period of time then this is side effect is not common. However, if the diarrhoea persists as soon as the renal diet makes up a certain percentage of the diet, addition of a high-fibre diet can resolve the problem. The quantity of food fed may need to be adjusted as the energy density of the new food may differ from the original.

Supporting the owner during the transition period of diet change is important, as the majority of affected animals are older, fastidious cats, some of which have very precise food preferences. A list of foods that should not be added to any commercial clinical diet can be useful for the owner.

Feeding habits of animals suffering from renal failure will alter, especially if the animal is uraemic and suffering from anorexia and nausea. Small, frequent meals can prove beneficial, as does feeding location and presentation. Food aversions can be a major problem with these animals, and if a clinical diet is flatly refused phosphate binders can prove to be useful.

Chronic renal failure in rabbits

See Chapter 14.

Key points

- Restricted protein levels are only recommended in patients with later stages of renal failure.

- Restricted salt levels are important. If the animal won't eat a commercial diet, consider the use of phosphate binders.
- Transitional changes can be difficult, and support from the veterinary practice may be required.

References

Allen TA, Polzin DJ, Adams LG. Renal disease. In: Hand MS, Thatcher CD, Remillard RL, Roudebush P, eds. *Small Animal Clinical Nutrition*, 4th edition. Topeka, KS: Mark Morris Institute, 2000, pp. 563–604.

Elliott DA. Nutritional management of chronic renal disease. *Waltham Focus* 2005; 15(1):14–19.

Elliott J, Rawlings JM, Markwell PJ, et al. Survival of cats with naturally occurring chronic renal failure: effect of dietary management. *J Small Anim Pract* 2000; 41:235–242.

Lane IF. Nutritional management of urinary tract conditions. In: Ettinger SJ, Feldman EC, eds. *Textbook of Veterinary Internal Medicine*, Vol. 1, 6th edition. St Louis, MO: Saunders Elsevier, 2005, pp584–586.

Plantinga EA, Everts H, Kastelein AMC, Beynen AC. Retrospective study of the survival of cats with acquired chronic renal insufficiency offered different commercial diets. *Vet Rec* 2005; 157:185–187.

Robertson JL, Goldschmidt M, Krionfeld DS, et al. Long-term renal responses to high dietary protein in dogs with 75% nephrectomy. *Kidney Int* 1986; 29:511–519.

32 Nutrition-Related Skin Disorders

The classification and diagnosis of nutrition-related skin disorders are initially based on a detailed dietary history and food evaluation. Dietary-induced skin problems include food intolerances, primary and secondary nutrient deficiencies, and nutrient toxicities (Roudebush et al. 2000). A diet history sheet can prove to be beneficial in obtaining all the necessary information (Appendix 1). A full dietary history needs to include specific commercial foods, all snacks and treats, supplements, chewable/palatable medications and vitamins, chew toys, human foods and any other food to which the animal may have access. The use of a food diary can also be helpful with obese and diabetic animals.

The terms 'food allergy' and 'food hypersensitivity' should be reserved for those adverse reactions to food that have an immunological basis. Food intolerance refers to adverse food reactions due to non-immunologic mechanisms. Dermatologists suggest that only 1–6% of all dermatoses seen in practice relate to adverse food reactions and that food allergies constitute 10–20% of allergic responses in dogs and cats (Roudebush et al. 2000; Figure 32.1). A full dermatological work-up is therefore required before a nutritional factor can be entirely confirmed. It is commonplace, however, for owners to self-diagnose their pet's food allergy or intolerance, even before seeing the veterinary surgeon.

The skin is the largest organ of the body and makes heavy demands on bodily nutrient supply. When factors become suboptimal it is usually the skin that becomes the first organ to demonstrate deterioration. The owner can easily detect signs of deterioration such as loss of coat sheen or coat shedding, and the coat can become greasy with scurf at the skin surface. Insufficiencies in the diet can be multifactorial and are shown in Table 32.1. Allergic reactions to dietary constituents can result in hives, which can sometimes arise when 'rich' feeds are suddenly introduced into the diet (Coatesworth 2006).

The Consulting Veterinary Nurse, First Edition. Nicola Ackerman.
© 2012 John Wiley & Sons, Ltd. Published 2012 by John Wiley & Sons, Ltd.

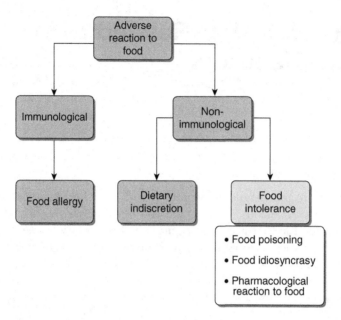

Figure 32.1 Flow diagram demonstrating different causes of adverse reactions to food.

Nurse clinics

The aim of nursing clinics and nutritional management is to:

- Help to avoid common food allergens
- Recommend a highly digestible diet where appropriate to limit the amount of undigested protein passing through to the gastrointestinal tract, which could provoke an allergic reaction
- Discuss with clients how to conduct an effective food trial, and the necessity to comply with strict restrictions
- Aid in diagnostic sampling if required.

The involvement of the veterinary nurse with dermatological cases is somewhat dependent on the veterinary practice. In many cases the role will be confined to discussing diet and parasite control. In some practices it can range from taking detailed histories, the performing of skin scrapes and blood sampling (see Chapter 4), and the administration of pharmaceuticals and immunotherapy agents. Discussion with the veterinary surgeons within the practice regarding the role of the dermatology nurse is important if you wish to expand this role.

Table 32.1 Deficiencies and their effect on the skin in the dog

Nutrient element	Function in relation to the skin and coat	Minimum canine requirement (per MJ)	Clinical signs of deficiency
Protein	Structure and pigment of keratinocytes and hair, component of sebum and sweat	9.6 g	Depigmentation of skin and hair, dry coat, hair loss
Lipids	Energy, precursors of eicosanoids, components of membrane phospholipids	3.3 g	Dull, dry coat, alopecia, greasy skin, pruritus
Linoleic acid	Maintenance of effective cutaneous barrier	0.66 g	Dry, scaly skin
Zinc	Metalloenzyme component, RNA and DNA polymerase cofactor	3.0 mg	Crusting/scaling of skin, erythema, alopecia
Copper	Melanin and keratinocyte synthesis	0.3 mg	Hypopigmentation and dry rough coat
Vitamin E	Antioxidant, stabiliser of cell membranes	1.8 IU	Scale, erythema, alopecia
Vitamin A	Cell growth and differentiation, keratinisation process	245.5 IU	Hyperkeratinisation, scaling, alopecia
Biotin	Metabolic enzyme cofactor	–	Facial alopecia and crusting
Riboflavin	Metabolic enzyme cofactor	0.15 mg	Dry, flaky dermatitis, swollen cracked lips
Niacin	Metabolic enzyme cofactor	0.72 mg	Pruritic dermatitis
Pyridoxine	Metabolic enzyme cofactor	0.07 mg	Dull, waxy coat and facial alopecia

Clinical nutrition

Fats

A common recommendation for atopic dermatitis is to supplement the diet with omega-6 and omega-3 (n-6 and n-3) essential fatty acids (EFAs). Dietary supplementation has been shown to normalise the cutaneous fatty acid profile and improve the clinical signs in dogs with seborrhoea. EFAs fulfil a number of roles in the body and skin. These include binding water into the stratum corneum, forming the epidermal permeability barrier, acting as antioxidants, and providing substrate for eicosaniods such as prostaglandin and leukotrienes. The omega-3 fatty acids compete with those of the omega-6 series for the same enzymes, so omega-3 supplementation will inhibit formation of arachidonic acid and its proinflammatory metabolites (Davenport and Reinhart 2000). The correct ratio of omega-6 to omega-3 fatty acids needs to be maintained within the diet. The recommended optimal levels are between 5:1 and 10:1 in the dog (Harvey 1996), but the understanding of dietary fatty acid ratios is less well defined in the cat and other species (Harvey 1996). Commonly administered fatty acid supplements include starflower/borage, evening primrose and corn oils, which are high in levels of omega-6 fatty acids. Cold-water sea fish, meat, linseed and soya contain omega-3 fatty acids. Dietary polyunsaturated fatty acids (PUFAs) have been also used in the management of certain inflammatory conditions, including allergic skin disease and arthritis.

Vitamins and minerals

Vitamin deficiencies are rarely diagnosed, and are unlikely to arise in the large proportion of animals that are fed a commercially balanced diet. Any deficiencies are more likely to be a consequence of a genetic enzyme defect, or an absorption problem. Vitamin deficiencies may occur in animals receiving a fat-restricted diet or having poor fat absorption. Some dietary components can also inactivate specific vitamins. For example, avidin in raw egg whites will bind biotin. Excessive amounts of the water-soluble vitamins can also be lost if the animal is suffering from polyuria. Vitamin A responsive dermatosis is entirely confined to cocker spaniels, and is a rare condition. The condition is characterised by focal areas of follicular plugging with accumulation of keratin. Daily doses of 10 000 IU of vitamin A are required to resolve these lesions (Lloyd 2001).

An absolute dietary deficiency of zinc deficiencies is considered to be rare. More commonly, there can be a relative deficiency due to interaction or an inability to utilise the ingested zinc. Absorption of zinc can be inhibited by iron, copper and calcium, and reduced by intestinal phytate and inorganic phosphate. Calcium, iron and copper all compete with zinc absorption. Animals that receive high levels of calcium in their diet are more likely to present with zinc deficiencies. These animals tend to be large or giant breeds, which receive over-supplementation of calcium during growth periods. Specific breeds such as Siberian huskies and Alaskan malamutes appear to be unable to absorb adequate quantities of zinc. Bull terriers can suffer from lethal acrodermatitis, a metabolic inability to utilise zinc. This can result in systemic signs such as emaciation, stunting and decreased immunocompetence. Zinc supplementation with oral zinc sulphate at 10 mg/kg body weight, or zinc methionate at 1.7 mg/kg body weight, once daily with food is the treatment of choice for the breed (Lloyd 2001). Supplementation for other breeds may be required for a period until any dermatological lesions resolve, provided that the animal is placed on a nutritionally balanced complete diet. Some may require lifelong supplementation.

Proteins

When designing or recommending an elimination diet, certain characteristics need to be taken into consideration. Carbohydrate from a limited number of sources is required, along with protein from a novel source. Excessive levels of protein should be avoided, and the protein present needs to have a digestibility greater than 87%. Hydrolysed protein can be used, as its digestibility is high. Digestibility is an important factor as free amino acids and small peptides make poor antigens. The diet needs to be free of additives and excessive levels of vasoactive amines, while still being nutritionally adequate for the animal's life stage and body score.

Hydrolysed diets are advantageous as they remove the absolute necessity of finding the primary causal agent of the food allergen. Hydrolysed diets work by reducing proteins in size through hydrolysis. When the hydrolysed protein is ingested, the body no longer recognises the protein as an antigen, and the allergic immune response is not initiated.

Carbohydrates

The use of carbohydrates in the diet also needs to be limited. In many elimination diets the a novel carbohydrate source is also used. Some of the many carbohydrates sources used include rice, potato and tapioca.

Feeding an elimination diet for dermatological or gastrointestinal disease

The main diagnostic method for nutritional adverse food reactions is dietary elimination trials. Either a commercial product or a homemade diet can achieve this purpose, but homemade diets are more likely to be nutritionally inadequate for maintenance requirements. Most homemade diets lack a source of calcium, EFAs, vitamins and other micronutrients. These diets also contain excessive levels of protein. If the owner insists on using a homemade diet, guidance on constructing a balanced diet is required from the veterinary practice.

In order to make a diagnosis of nutritional adverse food reactions, only the elimination diet can be used. The trial needs to last for a period of several weeks to months, and full dedication from the owner is required.

Elimination trials can prove to be extremely useful when diagnosing the causal nutritional agent in both dermatological and gastrointestinal disease. A strict elimination trial protocol must be adhered to, and the owner and anyone in contact with the animal needs to be aware of this (Figure 32.2). No foodstuffs other than the elimination food should be ingested over this period. This includes treats, flavoured vitamins, chewable/palatable medications; fatty acids supplements and chew toys. Advice must be clearly conveyed to the owner when discussing the use of an elimination food trial. Many owners do not realise that when feeding a

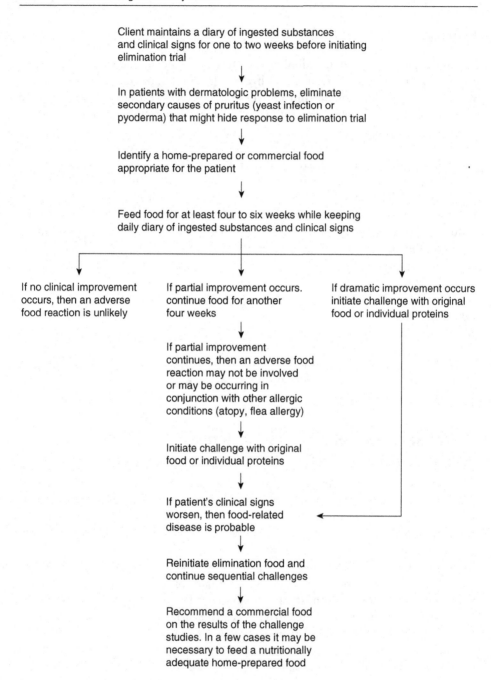

Figure 32.2 Diet protocol for elimination food trials (Roudebush et al. 2000).

specific protein (e.g. lamb) and carbohydrate-sourced diet, there should be no additional feeding of that specific protein (the lamb) in another form (e.g. processed).

For dermatological disease the patient is fed the controlled diet for 4–12 weeks. A shorter period of 2–4 weeks is usually satisfactory in gastrointestinal disease. The degree of clinical improvement during the elimination trial will be 100% only if food sensitivity is the sole causal agent. These trials are often difficult to interpret in dermatological disease, due to concurrent allergic skin disease. These patients may only partially respond to an elimination trial. Confirmation of a diagnosis can be made to an adverse food reaction when the clinical signs reoccur within 10–14 days after the animal has been given its original diet. Always give the client written instructions describing the requirements of the elimination trial, and feeding quantities.

Key points

- Good clear instructions are required for clients to refer to when completing a dietary trial, along with details of how to contact the clinic nurse if required
- Many dermatological conditions can only be managed, so support from the clinic nurse can aid in compliance and increasing welfare for the animal.

References

Coatesworth J. Essential fatty acids and canine atopy. *UK Vet Companion Anim* 2006; 63–64.

Davenport GM, Reinhart GA. Overview: the impact of nutrition on skin and hair coat. *Recent Advances in Canine and Feline Nutrition. Volume III, Iams Nutrition Symposium Proceedings*, 2000, pp. 3–21.

Harvey RG. Nutrition and skin disorders. In: Kelly N, Wills J, eds. *BSAVA Manual of Companion Animal Nutrition and Feeding*. Gloucester: BSAVA Publications, 1996, pp. 153–160.

Lloyd DH. Nutrition and the skin. Dermatology for veterinary nurses. *17th ESVD-ECVD Congress Veterinary Dermatology, Copenhagen*, 2001, pp. 145–153.

Roudebush P, Guilford WG, Shanley KJ. Adverse reactions to food 4. In: Hand MS, Thatcher CD, Remillard RL, Roudebush P, eds. *Small Animal Clinical Nutrition*, 4th edition. Topeka, KS: Mark Morris Institute, 2000, pp. 431–454.

33 Urinary Tract Disorders

Canine urolithiasis

Urolithiasis is considered to be a common disorder of the urinary tract in dogs. Clinical signs of urolithiasis may be the first indication of an underlying systemic disorder or defect in the structure or function of the urinary tract (Osborne et al. 2000). As with feline lower urinary tract disease (FLUTD), urolithiasis should be viewed not as a single disease process, but rather as a sequel of underlying abnormalities. Examination of the urolith composition will aid in determining the aetiology. A full dietary history is required, along with serum and urinalysis of the concentration of calculogenic mineral, crystallisation promoters and crystallisation inhibitors. Several types of urolith occur in dogs; each is discussed individually, as they require different treatments and managements (Table 33.1).

Urinary diets for dogs (and cats) can be divided in to those that promote dissolution through changing the pH of the urine and those that act by diluting the concentration of the urine. In all cases, dietary management should only commence once any obstruction (if present) has been resolved.

Nurse clinics

Canine urolithiasis is a disorder that needs long-term close monitoring because of the nature of reformation of crystals and stones. Dissolution and prevention of any future stones and crystals is the main aim of any clinic, and this can be achieved by:

- Decreasing the amount of calculogenic materials in the urine
- Increasing water intake
- Promoting an optimal pH (which is dependent on the urolith present)
- Helping the animal obtain its ideal weight and body condition score (BCS)
- Performing regular urine and blood sampling.

The Consulting Veterinary Nurse, First Edition. Nicola Ackerman.
© 2012 John Wiley & Sons, Ltd. Published 2012 by John Wiley & Sons, Ltd.

Table 33.1 Urolith formations and treatments, with urinary pH preferences

Type of urolith	Urinary pH during formation	Target urinary pH	Treatment
Struvite	Alkaline	5.9–6.3	Calculolytic diet or surgical removal
Calcium oxalate	Variable but usually acidic	7.1–7.7	Surgical removal
Ammonium urate	Acidic	7.1–7.7	Calculolytic diet and allopurinol
Cystine	Acidic	7.1–7.7	Calculolytic diet or surgical removal
Silicate	Usually acidic	7.1–7.7	Surgical removal

Source: Agar (2003).

Diagnostics

Blood sampling is a good indicator that the dog is receiving a low-protein diet, and can be used to check that the owner is solely feeding the diet, and not adding titbits or other foodstuffs to the daily portion. Further details on urine and blood sampling can be found in Chapter 4.

Clinical nutrition

The nutrition recommended can vary slightly depending on the stone or crystal present, and therefore any clinical nutritional recommendations for the specific stones are discussed separately.

Water

Water intake is a vital factor in dogs that have canine urolithiasis, or have a pre-disposition to it. The solute load of the diet greatly influences total water intake, in both dogs and cats. The use of a moist diet is preferred, and additional water can also be mixed in if required. Dogs can be encouraged to increase their consumption of water by placing more bowls of water around their environment to increase access. Bottled water, or water that has been pre-boiled or left to stand, will have little or no chlorine that can be detected by the dog. Some dogs will also play/eat ice cubes, especially useful in the warm weather, or like flavoured water. The use of filtered water in hard water areas can aid in reducing the intake of minerals.

Increased water consumption will increase the total volume of urine produced. Crystals precipitate out into the urine when supersaturation occurs. Urine becomes saturated when no more salt will dissolve within the fluid. Any additional salt or

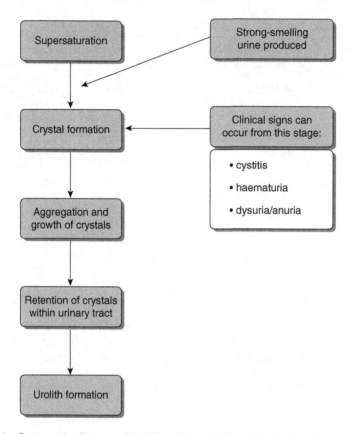

Figure 33.1 Systematic diagram of urolith and crystal formation in the urine.

decrease in the relative fluid volume will result in precipitation of the salt, and at this stage the urine is said to be supersaturated. Supersaturation of the urine is the initial stage of crystal urolith formation (Figure 33.1). Although urine supersaturation is fundamental for lithogenesis, the whole process is complex and multifactorial. Owners are recommended that the animal's urine should remain dilute and have no strong smell. Bitch's urine bleaches or kills the grass where urination commonly occurs, but this does not mean that crystals or uroliths are present.

Urinalysis should be done regularly, at least every 6 months once the animal is placed on a long-term urinary tract diet. Sediment analysis, pH and specific gravity are all good indicators of overall health. Fresh urine samples should be used when performing urinalysis. Samples obtained via cystocentesis should be used when obtaining samples for bacterial culture and sensitivity; this is especially important in dogs with suspected struvite or calcium phosphate uroliths. Urination should be encouraged as often as possible. Exercise in dogs can increase the frequency of urination.

Urate urolithiasis

Dalmatians have a high risk factor for recurrent urate uroliths, high enough that prophylactic therapy should be actively considered for this breed. Some texts state that Dalmatians are more susceptible as they lack the enzyme uricase, which converts uric acid to allantoin. Their urine therefore contains higher levels of urates than that of other breeds (Agar 2003). Other authors consider that uric acid metabolism is not caused by the absence of hepatic uricase (Buffington et al. 2004, Senior 1996), with enzyme levels being comparable to that in other breeds. The cause has been attributed to the impaired transport of uric acid into the hepatocytes, which may reduce the rate of hepatic oxidation. Another possibility is that the proximal renal tubules of Dalmatians reabsorb less and secrete more urate than the kidneys of other breeds of dogs (Buffington et al. 2004).

Clinical nutrition

Nutritional aims of dietary management of urate urolithiasis include:

- Restricting protein level
- Increasing the source of non-protein calories
- Promoting an alkaline urine pH.

Proteins

A diet designed to aid in urate urolithiasis should have restricted levels of proteins (1.6–2.2 g protein/100 kcal ME; Senior 1996), especially those proteins that are associated with larger amounts of nucleic acids, e.g. protein from muscle or organ tissues, as they contain purines. Milk proteins (casein) and eggs are suitable sources, as they contain a smaller amount of purines, but also have a high biological value, which is required when dietary protein levels are restricted.

Allopurinol needs to be added to the diet when dissolution of urate uroliths is required, though checking the diet manufacturer's guidelines is recommended. Allopurinol is a xanthine oxidase inhibitor, which reduces the rate of urate excretion into the urine. The dose rate should be 15 mg/kg by mouth twice a day, though this is dependent on the individual.

Carbohydrates and fats

Because of the restriction in protein levels, it is important that there is a sufficient supply of non-protein calories. This can imply a higher than normal fat content, and care should be given to the weight control of the animal. The level of fats also aids in obtaining the preferred urine pH.

Vitamins and minerals

As with any disease or disorder in which clinical symptoms include polyuria, the water-soluble vitamins should be supplemented. However, with urolithiasis vitamin C should not be supplemented, as it is a precursor of oxalate, and can predispose to its formation.

The alkalising agents used in these diets are commonly potassium citrate and calcium carbonate. If the target urinary pH is not reached, additional potassium citrate can be added to the diet at a starting dose rate of 50–100 mg/kg body weight by mouth twice a day, the amount given being adjusted according to effect (Senior 1996).

Struvite uroliths

Struvite uroliths are the most commonly occurring uroliths in dogs and in cats, although the incidence rate is decreasing. Infection-induced struvite uroliths are common in dogs. Antimicrobial therapy should be initiated alongside nutritional management, if urinalysis proves to be positive upon culturing. The bacteria present tend to be urease-producing staphylococci.

Clinical nutrition

Nutritional aims of dietary management of struvite uroliths include:

- Dissolution of uroliths within the bladder
- Preventing the formation of reoccurring uroliths or crystals
- Promoting an acidic urine pH.

Proteins
Restricted levels of protein are required (1.47 g protein/100 kcal ME), but a high biological value is needed. When protein levels are so restricted it is not advisable to feed this diet in the long term unless the digestibility of the proteins is high. The urine-acidifying substance in diets designed for struvite dissolution is DL-methionine, used at a dose rate of 0.5g/kg of diet.

Carbohydrates
The majority of calories obtained from the diet need to be obtained from a non-protein source. Thus, the carbohydrate and fat levels are increased in these diets.

Fats
Struvite diets can have very high fat levels (~26% DM), so much so that in some brands only tinned formulas are available. Feeding diets with such a high fat content to dogs with hyperlipidaemia, pancreatitis or even at-risk groups is contraindicated.

Vitamins and minerals
Decreased amounts of phosphorus (24 mg/100 kcal ME) and magnesium (3.3 mg/100 kcal ME) are present in the diet, as these are the constituents of the urolith. Sodium levels are often increased in these diets, in order to increase water intake (23.3 mg sodium/100 kcal ME). The antioxidants vitamin E and beta-carotene are often supplemented, as they help to reduce oxidative damage, and help combat urolithiasis. Vitamin C should not be supplemented, as it is a

precursor of oxalate, which can form when feeding diets designed for struvite dissolution.

Calcium oxalate uroliths

Calcium oxalate uroliths are the second most commonly occurring uroliths in the dog.

Clinical nutrition

Nutritional aims of dietary management include:

- Promoting an alkaline urinary pH
- Reducing the amounts of calcium, sodium and oxalates within the diet.

Protein
A low-protein diet is required. Levels of 1.6–2.2 g/100 kcal ME have been suggested in cases where calcium oxalate uroliths are present (Senior 1996).

Fats and carbohydrates
Non-protein calories are required in the diet, in order to prevent protein catabolism. Thus, levels of fats and carbohydrates are higher than normal. Weight management can be a problem in dogs that are predisposed to weight gain.

Vitamins and minerals
Neither vitamin D not vitamin C should not be supplemented into the diet. Vitamin D increases the absorption of calcium from the diet, whereas vitamin C acts as a precursor to oxalates. The levels of calcium in the diet should be restricted, but not reduced, as with levels of sodium. Sodium increases calcium excretion into the urine, and a dietary level of 0.1–0.2% sodium DMB or 45–55 mg sodium/100 kcal ME is recommended (Senior 1996).

Cystine uroliths

Cystine uroliths are uncommon in both cats and dogs, but arise due to a metabolic defect where the reabsorption of filtered cystine in the proximal tube is impaired (Bovee 1984). Once in the urine cystine is very insoluble, especially in acidic urine.

Clinical nutrition

Nutritional aims in the management of cystine uroliths include:

- Promoting an alkaline urine pH
- Reducing the amount of cystine produced by the body.

Protein

A low-protein diet is required (9–11% protein DMB), as this will aid in the reduction of the total daily excretion of cystine.

Carbohydrates and fats

Due to the low levels of protein in the diet, calories have to be obtained from these nutrients.

Vitamins and minerals

Low sodium levels are also required as sodium excretion can enhance cystine excretion. Low sodium in combination with low protein levels tends to increase the urine volume, which further decreases the urinary concentration of cysteine (Senior 1996). In order to create an alkaline urine pH, supplementation with potassium citrate (50–100 mg/kg body weight by mouth twice a day) is required, but care should be taken with animals with a history of GIT disease, as gastric disturbances can occur and even ulcerations at high doses.

Silicate uroliths

These uroliths are more commonly seen in male dogs (96%) than females (4%) (Osborne et al. 2000), probably because females can pass the smaller uroliths before they can induce clinical signs. Foods that contain large amounts of plant-derived materials are thought to be a predisposing factor for silicate uroliths; another factor is the consumption of soil.

Dietary management of dogs suffering from silicate uroliths involves prevention. Change of the diet to one that does not contain large amounts of plant-derived materials, and increases the volume of urine produced, are the main factors. There is debate about the urinary pH levels; alkalisation of the urine in order to increase the solubility of silica is unknown (Osborne et al. 1986).

Feeding a dog with urolithiasis

Nearly all diets aimed at dissolution or prevention of uroliths are high in fats, mainly because of the requirement for non-protein calories. Caution is required when transferring a dog over to these diets, particularly for dogs that are likely to gain weight, or those that are predisposed to hyperlipidaemia or pancreatitis. Diarrhoea can occur when high fat levels are fed, and combination with a high-fibre diet designed for urolith prevention may be required.

Calculolytic diets are only successful when fed alone. The addition of treats and home-cooked foods can undo the desired effect of the diet. It is equally important that the urolith analysis is correct. Stones of mixed composition are difficult to dissolve and surgical removal may be the treatment of choice. In dogs suffering from struvite urolithiasis, a blood sample analysis can be useful if you suspect that additional snacks or treats are being fed. In dogs being fed certain veterinary struvite dissolution diets, a low plasma urea concentration of less than 4 mmol/L (BUN 10 mg/dL) is found. A level higher than this suggests additional feeding.

Monitoring of dogs suffering from urolithiasis is vital. Urinalysis should be done at least every 6 months once dissolution has occurred. Preventive measures involve feeding a diet that promotes the correct urine pH, provide calories from a non-protein source and is relatively low in the salts that are the building blocks for the uroliths that the animal suffers from.

Key points

- Regular urinalysis whilst on the diet, including pH and microscopy is vital.
- Regular weight checks.
- Increase water intake as much as possible in all groups.
- Prevention in at-risk breeds outweighs cure.

Case study

An 11 year old Bichon Frise had undergone a cystotomy due to the presence of oxalate uroliths. In this case six points of action were recommended and undertaken:

1. Place on a prescription diet for uroliths, and avoid foods that contain milk, fish, cheese, etc.
2. Increase water consumption.
3. Take regular urine samples, checking urine pH (should be 7.1–7.7).
4. Measure blood calcium levels.
5. Culture urine for any bacterial infection.
6. Avoid obesity.

The dog was overweight (11.5 kg rather than the ideal 10 kg). Advice was given regarding exercise regimes and the dog was put on to a prescription veterinary diet. As the diet is low in protein and calories are obtained from the higher fat contents, digestion can be a problem in some dogs. In this case the dog's faeces were very soft, and this caused the owner concern, as hair was becoming matted around the dog's anus. The owner was recommended to mix in a high-fibre diet that can also be recommended for dogs suffering from uroliths. Adjustments in the proportions of diets were required until the diarrhoea was resolved. Urinalysis showed that even though the dog was on the correct diet, the urine pH was still at 5–6. Potassium citrate was required in order to help alkalinise the urine, at a dose rate of 50–150 mg/kg. A mid range of 1000 mg/day was administered, with urinalysis again being done regularly until optimal urine pH was achieved.

Table 33.2 Risk factors associated with increases in FLUTD cases

Age	Most commonly seen in cats between 1 and 10 years of age
Gender	Males and females have a similar risk of non-obstructive FLUTD. Prevalence of urethral obstruction is more common in males
Neuter status	Neutering in both males and females is associated with an increase in risk
Food	An increase in dry food consumption can increase risk factor
Weight	Excessive weight (obesity) will increase the risk of FLUTD
Water consumption	A decrease in water consumption can greatly increase the risk
Activity levels	Animals that have a more sedentary lifestyle are more likely to develop FLUTD
Weather conditions	Veterinary practices are more likely to see an increase in FLUTD cases when the weather is poor, possibly due to cats unwilling to urinate outdoors in wet weather

Feline lower urinary tract disease

Feline lower urinary tract disease (FLUTD) is becoming more prevalent, possibly because of an increase in the number of animals with higher risk factors (Table 33.2). FLUTD accounts for approximately 7% of feline cases presented to veterinary practices. FLUTD may result from a number of different aetiologies including infection, neoplasia, urolithiasis, neurological disorders, anatomical abnormalities and inflammatory conditions.

Urine is a composite of a complex solution of both organic and inorganic ions. Crystals can grow and form when an imbalance occurs in this complex solution. There are several factors that can cause these imbalances. Diet, decreased water consumption, urine pH alterations or relative lack of inhibitors of crystallisation can cause the solubility of a particular crystal to be exceeded. This result is crystal aggregation and growth. Clinical signs of FLUTD include haematuria, proteinuria, dysuria, polakiuria and/or urethral obstruction (Gunn-Moore 2000).

Nurse clinic

Dietary manipulation can aid in reducing the risk factors of uroliths, but there are many other factors that need to be taken in to consideration and addressed. Aims include:

- Take a full history of the environmental factors, and give advice regarding these factors
- Increase solubility of the products by obtaining a urinary pH that will dissolve any crystals that have formed in the urine, and aid in prevention of any further formation
- Eliminate or reduce the risk of supersaturation

- Increase the presence of inhibitors of crystallisation
- Aid the animal to obtain an ideal BCS if required
- Discuss strategies to reduce stressors for the cat.

Struvite crystals

Struvite crystals ($MgNH_4PO_4.6H_2O$) are commonly seen in cats suffering from FLUTD. Dietary recommendations for these cats include avoiding excessive dietary protein and avoiding excessive levels of the minerals that are used within the crystals (magnesium and phosphorus). Urinary pH needs to be acidic, as the crystals form in an alkaline environment. A range of 5.9–6.1 is ideal for dissolution, whereas 6.2–6.4 is recommended for prevention. The average urinary pH of a domestic cat consuming a natural diet (small rodents) is 6.3.

Acidifiers are used to prevent struvite uroliths. Cats receiving long-term dietary acidifiers can suffer from a transient negative potassium balance with phosphoric acid and ammonium chloride acidifiers. Long-term potassium depletion will stimulate ammonia synthesis at the same time as chronic metabolic acidosis. Acidifying therapeutic veterinary diets need to have potassium levels in excess of the United States National Research Council (NRC) minimum allowance of 0.6% DMB (Kirk 2000). The use of urinary acidifiers alongside an acidifying food is not recommended, as it can lead to metabolic acidosis. The alterations in pH may increase the solubility of some of the solutes within the urine, and in some cases decrease the solubility of others. This complex and competing interplay between nutritional requirements of the management of oxalate and struvite urolithiasis requires a careful selection in the long-term dietary control of FLUTD.

Oxalate crystals

Differences in the nutritional management of cats suffering from oxalate crystals include obtaining a less acidic urinary pH of 6.6–6.8. Citrate is commonly supplemented into diets specifically for cats suffering from oxalate crystals or uroliths. The citrate increases the urinary pH, and forms soluble complexes with the calcium, thus inhibiting calcium oxalate formation.

Clinical nutrition

Water

Water intake is a vital factor in cats with FLUTD or a predisposition to FLUTD. The solute load of the diet influences total water intake by a large factor. Use of a moist diet is preferred, and additional water can also be mixed in if required. A cat can be encouraged to increase its consumption of water by placing more bowls of water around its environment to increase access. The choice of type and size of water bowls used needs to be considered. Cats can be deterred from drinking fresh tap water because of its chlorine content. Bottled or pre-boiled water, or water that has been left to stand, will have little or no chlorine that the cat can detect. Further details are provided in Chapter 12.

Increases in water consumption will increase the total volume of urine produced. Crystals precipitate out into the urine when supersaturation occurs, i.e. when any additional salt or decrease in the relative fluid volume will result in precipitation of the salt. Supersaturation of the urine is the initial stage of crystal urolith formation (Figure 33.1). Although urine supersaturation is fundamental for lithogenesis, the whole process is complex and multifactorial. Owners are advised that the animal's urine should remain dilute and have no strong smell.

Urinalysis should be done on a regular basis, at least every 6 months. Sediment analysis, along with pH and specific gravity, are all good indicators of overall health. Idiopathic FLUTD can result in haematuria and proteinuria. Fresh urine samples should be used for urinalysis. Samples obtained via cystocentesis should be used for bacterial culture and sensitivity testing. Voided samples and those not examined immediately can give false positives for bacteria and crystalluria.

Protein

Excessive levels of protein need to be avoided in cases where struvite crystals and alkaline urine is present. High protein level can influence pH; a prime example of this is the difference in urine pH between cats and dogs. Cats have higher protein consumption than dogs, and therefore a higher urinary pH. Increasing the protein level in the diet also increases urinary calcium excretion, uric acid and oxalate excretion. Excess dietary protein should be avoided by feeding a food that contains 30–45% DM protein (Kirk 2000).

Fats

Diets that promote urinary tract health tend to have overall reduced mineral intake, a higher fat content and therefore increased energy density. When metabolised, fat produces the highest metabolic water contribution, which also benefits the animal. Because of their increased fat content some veterinary therapeutic diets are not available in a dry form. Obesity is a major risk factor for FLUTD, and a diet with a higher fat content may not be indicated in these circumstances.

Carbohydrates

Cats that suffer from FLUTD and are overweight need to be placed on an obesity diet. Many of these diets have a relatively high fibre content. The quantity of calcium being absorbed from the digestive system can be reduced by certain sources of dietary fibre. This can be beneficial with cats suffering from recurrent calcium oxalate urolithiasis.

Table 33.3 Recommended levels of minerals in commercial cat foods used for dissolution and prevention of struvite uroliths

Nutrient	% Dry matter		Caloric basis (g/100 kcal)	
	Prevention	Dissolution	Prevention	Dissolution
Phosphorus	0.5–0.9	0.5–0.8	0.11–0.24	0.11–0.17
Sodium	0.2–0.6	0.7–0.9	0.06–0.11	0.15–0.18
Magnesium	0.04–0.1	0.04–0.06	9–24	9–12

Table 33.4 Recommended levels of minerals in commercial cat foods used for dissolution of calcium-containing uroliths

Nutrient	% Dry matter	Caloric basis (g/100 kcal)
Calcium	0.5–0.8	0.11–0.2
Phosphorus	0.5–0.7	0.1–0.16
Sodium	0.1–0.4	0.03–0.1
Magnesium	0.04–0.1	0.018–0.020

Vitamins and minerals

Struvite precipitates form when the urine becomes supersaturated with magnesium, anionic phosphate and ammonium. Therapeutic diets avoid excess dietary magnesium, but low urinary magnesium concentrations have the potential to increase the risk of the formation of calcium-containing uroliths. This highlights the importance of regular urinalysis for a cat on a therapeutic urinary diet. The intake of magnesium and calcium also influences urinary phosphate concentrations (Tables 33.3 and 33.4).

Sodium is occasionally added to the diet in order to aid in increasing water intake. Increasing the salt content of the diet can aid in diuresis and lowers the urine specific gravity. Sodium does, however, increase calcium excretion in the urine, thus increasing the risk of calcium-based uroliths (e.g. oxalate). Increased sodium levels are also discouraged in older animals, because of the possibility of decreased renal function. A sodium level of 1.2% DMB has proved to present a health risk to cats when fed at this level in the long term (Sparkes 2006). Added antioxidants can help combat urolithiasis, by reducing oxidative cell damage.

Supplements

The use of nutraceuticals in cases of FLUTD is commonplace. Glycosaminoglycans (GAGs) and chondroitin are widely used to provide a protective lining to the bladder. In the healthy animal there is a GAG layer that lines the urothelium in the bladder, and contributes towards the protection of the bladder wall from substances present within the urine (e.g. crystals). Cats suffering from FLUTD can have a decreased excretion of urinary GAGs, and deficiencies in the GAG layer can contribute to urothelial damage, and ulceration and inflammation to the bladder wall (Sparkes 2006). The edges of the crystals can cause trauma to the lining of the bladder, resulting in haematuria. These types of nutraceuticals do not prevent recurrence of the crystals, but aid in prevention of some of the clinical signs. Evaluation of treatment should be made over a sufficient period of time (e.g. 3–6 months).

Feeding a cat with FLUTD

The choice of diet is dependent on two factors, the body condition of the animal and results of the urinalysis. Correct identification of the type of crystals present (if any) and the pH of the urine is necessary. Use of a diet that promotes urinary health tends to be aimed to prevent struvite formation. Use of these diets in cats with a predisposition to calcium oxalate uroliths may increase the risk of urolith formation. It should be noted that the prevalence of oxalate uroliths has been increasing, with a consequent decrease in struvite uroliths. A full dietary history of the cat is required (se Appendix 1), including any treats, supplements (especially if containing calcium) and whether or not the owner gives the cat milk. Treats and processed human food (processed meats) are high in mineral levels, such as phosphorus, and should be avoided.

Use of a moist diet is preferable, as is *ad libitum* feeding, but this feeding scenario might not be possible if the cat is overweight. When any animal consumes food, gastric acid is secreted and creates a temporary net acid loss from the body, and alkalisation of the urine. This is referred to as the postprandial alkaline tide. The alkaline tide is caused by secretion of bicarbonate into the blood by parietal cells of the stomach. A transient bicarbonisation is produced and increases urinary pH. Acidifiers in the diet will offset this increase in pH. If the diet is offered freely (*ad libitum*), the cat will eat little and often. These feeding habits result in a smaller but more prolonged alkaline tide. This can reduce the likelihood of struvite precipitate formation.

Recommendations should be given to clients about preventive measures in all cats. There are clear risk factors associated with FLUTD: some cannot be helped, such as age, breed and gender; others can, such as lifestyle and obesity. Neutering has a significant impact on the risk of bladder stones, the risk increasing sevenfold for oxalate stones and 3.5-fold for struvite stones (Lekcharoensuk et al. 2000). Educating the owner to ensure an adequate water intake and limiting weight gain after neutering is vital.

Reducing stress in cats

The influence of behavioural responses in the cat has been widely linked to the occurrence of FLUTD. Clients need to be made aware of this link and given appropriate advice in order to help their cat. Many cats can be presented to the veterinary practice for behavioural problems with inappropriate urination, but FLUTD needs to be ruled out before the instigation of behavioural treatments.

- Food intake disorders (anorexia or overfeeding)
- Overgrooming (bald areas) or undergrooming (matted or soiled fur)
- House soiling, inappropriate urination or defecation
- Decreasing levels of activity, increased resting or feigned sleep
- Appearing withdrawn (reduced desire to play or interact), hiding
- Extreme vigilance and heightened startle response
- Defensive aggression towards people and other cats in the household, e.g. hissing
- Increased dependency or social withdrawal (dependent on personality type)
- Changes in patterns of behaviour, e.g. spending a more significant amount of time indoors, irrespective of normal seasonal changes
- Urine spraying.

Understanding these sometimes very subtle signs can be very difficult for clients. In multi-cat households the presence of other cats can be the main cause, and removal of the cause is impossible. Owners need to be supported in order to make changes to the household to help the stressed animal. There need to be sufficient resources in the household in order to reduce competition for them. This means that more litter trays, food bowls and water bowls are required than there are cats within the household. All of these resources need to be kept separate from one another, as cats do not like to eat, drink and eliminate in the same area.

Key points

- Increase water intake, and thus urinary dilution. Urine specific gravity is a more important factor than urine pH.
- Perform regular urinalysis, even once dissolution has been achieved. It is also be recommended that a full blood haematology and biochemistry should be done on a regular basis, due to the link between FLUTD and renal failure in older cats.
- Educate clients to take preventive measures against the formation of urinary calculi throughout a cat's life, starting from a young age.
- Maintain a urinary pH of 6–6.5 in healthy cats, where dissolution is not required.

Case study

A 6 year old male neutered cat was presented with haematuria and dysuria. The cat was grossly overweight (9.8 kg; ideal weight 5 kg), and had a BCS of 5/5.

Microscopy of the urine showed large amounts of struvite crystals and erythrocytes. Blood samples were taken to confirm renal function before placing the cat on NSAIDs. A course of antibiotics was also implemented. The cat was placed on a weight reduction diet, which also aided in the dissolution of the struvite crystals. Water consumption also had to be dramatically increased in this cat, and thus a moist diet was use along with suggestions in Chapter 12. The cat's activity levels also needed to be increased. The owner was told to place the cat's food in different places so that it had to go find the food, and toys were also introduced.

The cat was monitored regularly for the weight loss, and urinalysis routinely carried out every 6 months.

Urolithasis in rabbits

See Chapter 14.

References

Agar S. *Small Animal Nutrition*. Edinburgh: Butterworth Heinemann, 2003.

Bovee KC. Genetic and metabolic diseases of the kidney. In: Bovee KC, ed. *Canine Nephrology*. Media, PA: Harwal Publications, 1984, pp. 339–354.

Buffington T, Holloway C, Abood S. *Manual of Veterinary Dietetics*. St Louis, MO: Elsevier Saunders, 2004.

Gunn-Moore DA. *Update on Feline Lower Urinary Tract Disease*. Watford: Ceva Animal Health Ltd, 2000.

Kirk CA. Dietary salt and FLUTD: risk or benefit? *Proceedings of the 20th Annual ACVIM Forum* 2000; 553–555.

Lekcharoensuk C, Lulich JP, Osborne CA. Association between patients related factors and risk of calcium oxalate and magnesium ammonium phosphate urolithiasis in cats. *J Am Vet Med Assoc*, 2000; 217:520–525.

Osborne CA, Clinton CW, Kim KM. Etiopathogenesis, clinical manifestations and management of silica urolithiasis. *Vet Clin North Am Small Anim Pract* 1986; 16:185–207.

Osborne CA, Bartges JW, Lulich JP, et al. Canine urolithiasis. In: Hand MS, Thatcher CD, Remillard RL, Roudebush P, eds. *Small Animal Clinical Nutrition*, 4th edition. Topeka, KS: Mark Morris Institute, 2000, pp. 605–688.

Senior DF. Urolithiasis – a nutritional perspective. In: Kelly N, Wills J, eds. *BSAVA Manual of Companion Animal Nutrition and Feeding*. Gloucester: BSAVA Publications, 1996, pp. 188–197.

Sparkes A. Urolithiasis in cats: optimum management to prevent recurrence. *Vet Rev* 2006; 115:20–28.

Appendix 1 Diet History Sheet

Animal's information

Animal's name: Date:
Client name:
Current weight: Optimal weight: BCS:
Breed: Age: Sex: M/F N/E
Current diseases:
Medications:
Activity level of the animal:
Quantity of exercise the animal receives:
Appetite levels:

Dietary information

Current brand of food being fed:
Is the diet: moist/dry/mixed   complete/complementary
Quantities at each meal:
Number of meals:
Treats being fed, and quantity:
Table/human foods:

  Breakfast
  Lunch
  Dinner
  Between meals

Food covering medications:
Food additives:
Vitamins/supplements:
Palatable medications:

The Consulting Veterinary Nurse, First Edition. Nicola Ackerman.
© 2012 John Wiley & Sons, Ltd. Published 2012 by John Wiley & Sons, Ltd.

Owner and environmental information

How many pets are in the household?
Do they feed together?
Where is the pet fed?
Is there competition for food?
Does the animal have access to other pet's food (neighbour)?
Who feeds the animal?
Are there other people in the household?
Does the animal scavenge?
Is more than one animal fed out of each feeding dish?
Is the food measured out?

Appendix 2 Unit Conversion Tables

Mass (weight)

1 kg	=	2.204	lbs (pounds
1 ounce (oz, avoirdupois)	=	28.3	g (grams)
1 ounce (oz, troy)	=	31.1	g (grams)
1 lb	=	16	oz (ounces)
		454	g (grams)
1 stone	=	14	lbs (pounds
		6.35	kg
1 hundredweight (cwt)	=	112	lbs (pounds)
		8	stones
		50.8	kg
1 ton (imperial or UK)	=	2240	lbs (pounds)
		160	stones
		20	hundredweight (cwt)
		1016	kg
1 ton (short ton or US)	=	2000	lbs (pounds)
		907	kg
1 tonne (metric)	=	2204	lbs (pounds)

The Consulting Veterinary Nurse, First Edition. Nicola Ackerman.
© 2012 John Wiley & Sons, Ltd. Published 2012 by John Wiley & Sons, Ltd.

Volume

1 imperial fluid ounce(fl oz)	=	28.41	mL
1 imperial pint	=	20	fluid ounces (fl oz)
		0.568	litres
1 imperial quart	=	1.137	litres
1 imperial (UK) gallon	=	160	fluid ounces (fl oz)
		8	pints
		4	quarts
		4.546	litres
1 US fluid ounce (US fl oz)	=	29.6	mL
1 US pint	=	16	US fluid ounces (US fl oz)
		0.473	litres
1 US quart	=	0.946	litres
1 US gallon	=	128	US fluid ounces (US fl oz)
		8	US pints
		1.785	litres

Temperature conversion

Celsius (°C) °C = 5/9 (°F-32)	Fahrenheit (°F) °F = 9/5 (°C) + 32
−273.15	−459.67
−40	−40
−17.78	0
0	**32**
10	50
20	68
30	86
35	95
36.0	**96.8**
36.5	**97.7**
37.0	**98.6**
37.5	**99.5**
38.0	**100.4**
38.5	**101.3**
39.0	**102.2**
39.5	**103.1**
40.0	**104.0**
40.5	**104.9**
41.0	**105.8**
41.5	**106.7**
42.0	**107.6**
42.5	**108.5**
43.0	**109.4**
43.5	**110.3**
44.0	**111.2**
44.5	**112.1**
45.0	**113.0**
45.5	**113.9**
46.0	**114.8**
50	122
60	140
70	158
80	176
90	194
100	**212**
150	302
200	392
300	572
400	752
500	932
600	1112
700	1292
800	1472
900	1652
1000	1832

Glossary

Aerophagia   The habit of swallowing air while eating.

Anthropomorphism   The attribution of human-based perceptions to an animaal's needs or preferences.

Availability (bioavailability)   The degree to which a drug or nutrient becomes available to the target tissue after administration or consumption.

Azotaemia   Presence of excess nitrogen-containing compounds in the blood.

Bacterial translocation   Bacteria moving from one place (gut lumen) into another (bloodstream) because of mucosal breakdown.

Biological value   A measure of the proportion of protein absorbed from the diet that becomes incorporated into the proteins of an animal's body.

Borborygmus   Noises from the abdomen associated with gas or fluids passing through the intestinal tract.

Cachexia   A profound state of general ill health and starvation, characterised by severe body wasting.

Cholangiohepatitis   Inflammation of the biliary ducts and liver.

Coprophagy   Habit of eating faeces.

Cystocentesis   A procedure where a sample of urine is removed by means of a needle inserted into the urinary bladder through the abdomen.

Dystocia   Difficulty in giving birth.

Gastrocolic reflex   This reflex is responsible for the urge to defecate following a meal. It involves an increase in motility of the colon in response to stretch in the stomach and by-products of digestion in the small intestine.

Haematuria   The presence of blood in the urine.

Hyperglycaemia   The presence of too much glucose in the blood. A symptom of uncontrolled diabetes.

Hyperlipidaemia   The presence of too much lipid (fat) or lipoproteins in the blood.

Hypertension   A chronic condition in which the blood pressure in the arteries is too high.

Immunocompetence   The ability to develop an immune response after exposure to an antigen.

The Consulting Veterinary Nurse, First Edition. Nicola Ackerman.
© 2012 John Wiley & Sons, Ltd. Published 2012 by John Wiley & Sons, Ltd.

Melaena   Presence of digested blood in the faeces, resulting in black tarry stools.

Morphometry   Measurement of the structures and parts of organisms.

Neutrophils   A type of white blood cell that forms part of the immune system.

Ossification   Bone tissue formation.

Osteoclasts   Cells that absorb bone, allowing for the deposition of new bone and maintenance of bone strength.

Pica   Craving or eating unusual substances.

Steatorrhoea   The presence of fats in the faeces.

Tenesmus   The act of straining to pass urine or faeces.

Uroliths   Stones formed in the bladder as a result of oversaturation of urine with crystals.

Index

The Consulting Veterinary Nurse, First Edition. Nicola Ackerman.
© 2012 John Wiley & Sons, Ltd. Published 2012 by John Wiley & Sons, Ltd.

Printed in the United States
By Bookmasters